death is
but a
dream

# death is but a dream

## Finding Hope and Meaning at Life's End

### Christopher Kerr, MD, PhD

*with* Carine Mardorossian, PhD

Avery ✳ an imprint of Penguin Random House ✳ New York

AVERY

an imprint of Penguin Random House LLC
penguinrandomhouse.com

Grateful acknowledgment is made to reprint from the following:
"A Change of Address" by Dónall Dempsey. Reprinted with permission of Dónall Dempsey.

*The Poems of Emily Dickinson*, edited by Thomas H. Johnson, Cambridge, MA: The Belknap Press
of Harvard University Press. Copyright © 1951, 1955 by the President and Fellows of Harvard
College. Copyright © renewed 1979, 1983 by the President and Fellows of Harvard College.
Copyright © 1914, 1918, 1919, 1924, 1929, 1930, 1932, 1932, 1935, 1937, 1942 by Martha
Dickinson Bianchi. Copyright © 1952, 1957, 1958, 1963, 1965 by Mary L. Hampson.

"Stitches," words and music by Teddy Geiger, Danny Parker, and Daniel Kyriakides.
Copyright © 2015 Music of Big Deal, TG WorldWide Publishing, The Family Songbook, Danny
Clementine Music, Hold The Dog, and Megahouse Music. All rights administered by Words &
Music, a division of Big Deal Music, LLC. All rights reserved. Used by permission.
Reprinted by permission of Hal Leonard LLC.

Most Avery books are available at special quantity discounts for bulk purchase
for sales promotions, premiums, fund-raising, and educational needs.
Special books or book excerpts also can be created to fit specific needs.
For details, write SpecialMarkets@penguinrandomhouse.com.

Library of Congress Cataloging-in-Publication Data

Names: Kerr, Christopher, MD, author. | Mardorossian, Carine M., author.
Title: Death is but a dream: finding hope and meaning at life's end /
Christopher Kerr, MD, PhD; with Carine Mardorossian.
Description: New York: Avery, an imprint of Penguin Random House LLC, 2020. |
Includes bibliographical references and index. | Summary: "The first book to explore the
meaningful dreams and visions that bring comfort as death nears." —Provided by publisher.
Identifiers: LCCN 2019038405 (print) | LCCN 2019038406 (ebook) |
ISBN 9780525542841 (hardcover) | ISBN 9780525542858 (epub)
Subjects: LCSH: Death in dreams. | Dream interpretation. | Death—Psychological aspects.
Classification: LCC BF1099.D4 K47 2020 (print) | LCC BF1099.D4 (ebook) | DDC 155.9/37—dc23
LC record available at https://lccn.loc.gov/2019038405
LC ebook record available at https://lccn.loc.gov/2019038406

Printed in the United States of America
1   3   5   7   9   10   8   6   4   2

Book design by Lorie Pagnozzi

The bookends of my life have been strong women. A secret conspiracy of old and young women, ones who raised me and ones whom I have raised. This book is for them.

To my grandmother Violet, who fought through the hardships of her times and emerged ennobled by the scars. She did not suffer foolish men, neither gladly nor at all. To her grandchildren, she was full of humor and great humanity.

To my mother, Shirley, whose eyes can never look beyond the needs of others, and who rebels as much as she achieves. Thank you for laughing out loud when my first grade teacher said of me "Don't expect too much." Then and now, you have made all things possible and the world a wonder.

To my daughter Bobbie, who at age three pointed to the moon and asked, "Did you make dat?" I said no, and you were saddened. Then I showed you something better—a horse. As you touched his mane, he touched your heart, and together you began a journey toward your life's passion and purpose. Some days I like you better on a horse, but on all days—now and forever—I will love you to "dat" moon and back.

To my daughter Maddie, who has taught us the real prize doesn't go to the winner of the race, or of any contest, for that matter. There is no prize for goodness. Indeed, the good ones simply become our heroes. You are mine.

No one ever had to tell me you were strong women.
There was never a need. I always knew.

# contents

*✳*

# introduction

In examining disease, we gain wisdom about anatomy and
physiology and biology. In examining the person with disease,
we gain wisdom about life.

—OLIVER SACKS

Tom was only forty when he arrived at Hospice Buffalo with
end-stage AIDS. Unlike most of my patients, he was not surrounded by loved ones. Not a soul came to visit, ever. He was
rather stoic, so I wondered if the absence of visitors was his
choice rather than an indicator of his loneliness. Maybe that
was his way of refusing to give death an audience.

I was puzzled but, wanting to respect his privacy, did not inquire. Tom's emaciated body showed traces of once-chiseled
muscles. He had kept fit and was still quite young, which gave
me hope. In light of his age and physical conditioning, I thought
that his body would be more likely to respond positively to life-
prolonging treatment. Not long after he was admitted, I went to
the nurse's station and decreed, "I think we can buy Tom some
time. IV antibiotics and fluids should do it."

The charge nurse, Nancy, had been at Hospice Buffalo for
much longer than I had. She knew her job, and everyone looked

up to her. She was also not one to mince words. Still, her response took me by surprise: "Too late. He's dying."

I said, "Oh really?"

She replied, "Yep. He's been dreaming about his dead mother."

I chuckled awkwardly—equal parts disbelief and defensiveness. "I don't remember that class from medical school," I said.

Nancy did not miss a beat. "Son, you must have missed a lot of classes."

I was a thirty-year-old cardiology fellow finishing my specialty training while working weekends at Hospice Buffalo to pay the bills. Nancy was an exceptional veteran nurse who had limited patience for young, idealistic doctors. She did what she always did when someone was out of their depth—she rolled her eyes.

I went about my business, mentally running through all the ways modern medicine could give Tom another few weeks or even months. He was riddled with infection, so we administered antibiotics. Because he was also severely dehydrated, I asked for a saline drip. I did all I could do as a doctor to prolong his life, but within forty-eight hours, Tom was dead.

Nancy had been right in her estimation of where he was on the downward slope. But how could she have known? Was it just pessimism, the numbing effect of having watched so many people die? Was she truly using a patient's dream as a predictor of life-span? Nancy had worked in hospice for more than two decades. She was tuned in to aspects of dying I knew nothing about: its subjective dimensions. How patients experienced illness, particularly dying, had mostly been ignored throughout my training as a doctor.

Like many physicians, I'd never considered that there might be more to death than an enemy to be fought. I knew about blind intervention—doing everything possible to keep people conscious and breathing—but had little regard for the way any given individual might wish to die, or for the unavoidable truth that ultimately death is inevitable. Because it had not been part of my medical education, I failed to see how the subjective experience of dying could be relevant to my role as a doctor.

It was ultimately the remarkable incidence of pre-death dreams and visions among my dying patients that made me realize how significant a phenomenon this was, both at a clinical and a human level. As a hospice doctor, I have been at the bedsides of thousands of patients who, in the face of death, speak of love, meaning, and grace. They reveal that there is often hope beyond cure as they transition from a focus on treatment to notions of personal meaning. As illness advances, grace and grit collide and bring new insight to those dying and their loved ones, insight that is often paradoxically life-affirming. This experience includes pre-death dreams and visions that are manifestations of this time of integration and coming into oneself. These are powerful and stirring experiences that occur in the last days or hours of life and that constitute moments of genuine insight and vivid re-centering for patients. They often mark a clear transition from distress to acceptance, a sense of tranquility and wholeness for the dying. Patients consistently describe them as "more real than real," and they are each as unique as the individual having them.

These end-of-life experiences are centered on personal histories, self-understanding, concrete relationships, and singular events. They are made of images and vignettes that emanate from each person's life experiences rather than from abstract preoccupations with the great beyond. They are about a walk in the woods relived alongside a loving parent, car rides or fishing trips taken with close family members, or seemingly insignificant details such as the texture or color of a loved one's dress, the feel of a horse's velvety muzzle, or the rustling sound of a cottonwood's shimmering leaves in the backyard of a childhood home. Long-lost loved ones come back to reassure; past wounds are healed; loose ends are tied; lifelong conflicts are revisited; forgiveness is achieved.

Doctors owe it to their patients to incorporate this awareness into their practice. End-of-life experiences ought to be recognized as evidence of the life-affirming and inspiring resilience of the human spirit that drives them. They are proof of humanity's built-in, natural, and profoundly spiritual capacity for self-sustenance and self-healing, grace and hope. They help restore meaning at end of life and assist in reclaiming dying as a process in which patients have a say. They also benefit those left behind, the bereaved, who get relief from seeing their loved ones die with a sense of peace and closure.

This subjective experience of dying is also a powerful reminder that beauty and love in human existence often manifest themselves when we least expect it. The patients who summon up comforting processes at life's end are beset by symptoms of a failing body over which they have limited control. They are at their most frail and vulnerable, existing within suffering states of aching bones and hunger for air. Catheters, IVs, and pills may now be part of their every day, sometimes literally functioning as extensions of their bodies under the daily medical management that is their new and irreversible lot. They may experience various degrees of cognitive, psychological, and spiritual dissonance. Yet even as the inexorable march of time is taking its toll on their bodies and minds, many also have pre-death dreams and visions in the context of which they display remarkable awareness and mental sharpness.

Herein truly lies the paradox of dying: patients are often emotionally and spiritually alive, even enlightened, despite a precipitous physical deterioration. The physical and psychological toll of dying may be undeniable, but it is also what makes the emotional and spiritual changes brought about by end-of-life experiences border on the miraculous. Doing justice to end-of-life experiences means accounting for this paradox, one in which death and dying transcend physical decline and sadness to include spiritual awakening, beauty, and grace. Or, as the title character in the acclaimed *Tuesdays with Morrie* puts it, "Aging is not just decay, you know. It's growth. It's more than the negative that you're going to die." This is also true of the dying process, which often functions as a summing up, culmination, and capstone, an opportunity to recognize and celebrate our humanity in all its complexity and dignity rather than just as an ending.

My hope is that this book will inform and empower patients nearing death, as well as their families and caretakers. It brings to life the stories of the exceptional people who've been willing to share their dreams, thoughts, and feelings as they approached their final transition. It is meant for those who will, sooner or later, "cross the threshold of eternity," which is to say, everyone. It is *about* living and *for* the living.

These are brave individuals such as Kenny, a retired funeral home director and father of five children, who, right before his death at age seventy-six, was visited by the beloved mother he had lost when he was only six years old. As death neared, he appeared as a little boy in his dreams, and could hear his mother's soothing voice uttering the words "I love you" again and again. He even reported being able to smell the distinct aroma of her perfume in his hospital room.

Or ninety-one-year-old Deb, a retired retail worker at a department store, who eight days before passing from ischemic heart disease had "extremely comforting" visions of six deceased family members in her room, including her father, who "was waiting for me." A day later, she saw herself being driven away by her childhood friend Leonard as her deceased aunt Martha exhorted her to "let go."

Another patient, Sierra, at twenty-eight and facing the unbearable thought of her four-year-old boy becoming motherless, was understandably in denial about the severity of her condition. The cancer hospital had sent her to hospice "to be more comfortable," a metaphorical turn of phrase she interpreted literally with all the sanguineness of youth. "I am going to beat this," she whispered to our confused staff mere days before her death. A vision of her deceased grandfather telling her he didn't want her to suffer anymore finally brought acceptance and gave her and her grieving family the strength to let go. She no longer feared her own nonexistence and died peacefully in her mother's arms.

And then there was Jessica, who, at thirteen, taught me how to come to terms with the inconceivable, the passing of a child. When I asked her what the dreams she'd been having meant to

her, she simply responded, "That I am loved. I will be fine."
There are times when it takes the innocence of a child to guide
us through the unbearable.

⊰≮⊱

The prejudices of present-day medical training have caused an
inability to see dying as anything but failure, and they compromise the self-soothing power of patients' end-of-life experiences.
Simply put, doctors often see end-of-life experiences as irrelevant to their craft. Medical students and physicians are trained
to dismiss anything that cannot be measured, imaged, biop-
sied, or removed.

It's also true that the medical profession is more comfortable
with questions of the brain than with questions of the mind, so
the words and experiences of the dying are easily dismissed as
the ramblings of people who are cognitively impaired or possibly suffering the side effects of medications. Our current medical model reflects a limited view of the totality of the dying
experience.

In the evolution from treating illness to caring for the dying,
medical staff should lead the way instead of denying or merely
medicating these powerful end-of-life experiences. Patients
and their families should be encouraged to speak about them
openly with their medical care providers. This helps enhance
patients' mental well-being, and it helps doctors dispense better
care. Managing symptoms medically should include promoting
dying patients' psychological and spiritual well-being, as well as
preserving patient dignity at life's end.

How can such a careful balance be achieved? I believe that no one other than the patient can or should answer this question. Few researchers have directly asked those who are nearing death exactly what it is they are experiencing, what their dreams and visions mean to them, and how they affect their physical and mental states.

Again, this is largely because medical training is about defying death. Having myself been there and done that with nurse Nancy and our patient Tom, I knew that to convince my colleagues to change their ways, we would have to translate end-of-life experiences into a language they understood, the language of evidence-based research. So we conducted structured interviews to provide said evidence. We provided quantifiable data, lots of it. But I didn't know then what I know now, namely that it takes much more than data and statistics to produce the kind of revolution in our treatment of dying that would help patients and their families.

This book is therefore a plea: we need to bring doctors back to the bedside, to their roots as comforters of the dying rather than as mere technicians trying to extend life at all costs. This includes examining end-of-life experiences in a caregiving framework and accepting them as medically important. Studies have shown that despite the value and positive significance of these experiences, patients are reluctant to discuss them due to a fear of ridicule and questions regarding their medical legitimacy. And because many physicians simply avoid addressing them, this widespread inattention further isolates the dying. Patients' inner experiences matter to them; therefore, they should matter to doctors. An awareness of their clinical significance and universality will close the gap that currently exists between the care given and the care needed.

The acceleration of the science of medicine has obscured its art, and medicine, always less comfortable with the subjective, has been more concerned with disproving the unseen than revering its meaning. Gaining access to the human emotions that are not available to science therefore means turning to other disciplines. This is especially true of dying, the time when nature assumes its rightful role and medicine can no longer defy death. In the prescient words of the sixteenth-century philosopher Montaigne, "If you know not how to die, never trouble yourself; Nature will in a moment fully and sufficiently instruct you; she will exactly do that business for you; take you no care for it." He was right. When we do not overly medicalize the process of dying and instead dignify and validate near-death experiences in all their physical and spiritual dimensions, dying becomes less about death than about life's resilience.

The richest, most thoughtful and resonant discussions on dying have come from the humanities—from writers, poets, and philosophers as far back as ancient Greece—and from Buddhist and Islamic texts to accounts from China, Siberia, Bolivia, Argentina, India, and Finland. Meaningful pre-death dreams and visions have been recognized in the religious and sacred traditions of Native Americans and other indigenous peoples around the world. They are mentioned in the Bible, in Plato's *Republic*, and in medieval writings such as the fourteenth-century mystic Julian of Norwich's *Revelations of Divine Love*. They show up in Renaissance paintings and in Shakespeare's *King Lear*. They appear in nineteenth-century American and British novels, in T. S. Eliot's poetry, and last but not least in the Dalai Lama's meditations on death. If anything, the medicalization of death has obscured a language that has always been available to make sense of our finitude and that has been integral to humanity's cultural need to maintain connection with the departed.

In contrast to humanist thinkers' long-standing obsession with the subjective aspects of dying, anthropologists, sociologists, psychoanalysts, scientists, and medical professionals have examined end of life in detail only since the beginning of the twentieth century. These disciplines aim mostly to describe and prove hypotheses in a more or less objective fashion. There is no doubt a place for all of these perspectives in our approach to dying, but the differences are crucial when trying to redress the overmedicalization of mortality in our contemporary lives. It explains why patients themselves, as well as their caretakers, are more drawn to the imaginative and creative arts when it comes to making sense of their end-of-life journey.

William Barrett, a professor of physics at the Royal College of Science for Ireland in Dublin, appears to have written the first scholarly book on the subject in 1926. *Deathbed Visions* was based on the observations of his wife, an obstetrician, who described the visions of a woman who died in childbirth. But the study of the phenomenon there too is primarily focused on proving a hypothesis—whether the visions are of the afterlife or the paranormal—often at the exclusion of the patient perspective, the only voice that matters. In the West, end-of-life dreams and visions have more recently been discussed as evidence of phenomena ranging from the neuronal workings of a dying brain to the consequences of oxygen deprivation, an approach that has not accounted any more than previous ones for the view from the bed, the one that matters.

In light of the limitations of science when it comes to representing the subjective dimensions of dying, it is not surprising then that Atul Gawande, surgeon by day and public health author by night, chose to reference a literary text to introduce his masterful exploration of aging, death, and medicine. *Being Mortal* begins with his reading of a short story by novelist Leo Tolstoy, a literary text that recounts the suffering of the dying protagonist Ivan Ilyich. Similarly, the neurosurgeon Paul Kalanithi's posthumous memoir about living and dying with cancer derives its haunting title, *When Breath Becomes Air*, from a literary source, a poem titled "Caelica 83" (1633), which was written by an Elizabethan author named Baron Brooke Fulke Greville. And last but not least, when Nina Riggs, a poet and mother of two, received a terminal diagnosis of breast cancer at the age of thirty-seven, she too turned to literature to make "the experience of living with death in the room every day one that everyone can relate to."

Again and again, patients, as well as their caregivers, turn to poems, plays, or novels to make sense of their mortality. At a time when bodily symptoms and decline seem to overtake otherworldly considerations, it is often fiction and creative works rather than nonfictional representations of reality that speak to the terminally ill in profound and resonant ways. Dying patients, maybe more than anyone, yearn for insight into their end-of-life experience, an experience that seems first to transcend reason but that ultimately brings another level of understanding.

⸎

In 2015, I gave a TEDx Buffalo Talk about what it meant to have gathered data based on the direct testimonies of dying patients.

On the heels of that, the work was featured in the *New York Times*, *Huffington Post*, *Psychology Today*, *Scientific American Mind*, and the *Atlantic Monthly*. Then a documentary film crew approached us, and within the first week, the teaser for their film attracted more than six hundred thousand views on Facebook. It was clear that the public at large was drawn to this subject in a way that doctors were not. This discrepancy was emblematic of the gap between the perceived and the actual needs of patients and their loved ones.

The feedback was simply overwhelming; testimonials from families and friends who sat vigil at the bedside of dying loved ones and bore witness to end-of-life dreams and visions clearly revealed a need for such experiences to be addressed in a care-giving framework.

As hospice work demonstrates again and again, when the patient is kept comfortable and otherwise left to follow the natural course of things, death becomes more enlightening than a simple pulling down of the shades. The tragedy of human existence is not the fact of death or suffering or the inability to defeat them. It is the inability to rethink dying as anything other than the "dimming of the light." It is, in the philosopher Alan Watts's words, "that when such facts are present, we circle, buzz, writhe, and whirl, trying to get the 'I' out of the experience." To me, rewriting the "I" of the patient into the shrouded story of humanity's finitude means making the subjective experience of dying a crucial part of how I medically treat my patients.

It has become easier to live longer but harder to die well. We have lost our way with dying and with death. Most Americans want to die at home in the care of loved ones, yet many die in institutions, often alone or in the care of strangers. The death people wish for often becomes the one they fear, a sanitized and undignified one. Amid the current madness of medical excess, there is a need for spiritual renewal that medicine alone cannot address. By exploring the nonphysical experience of dying, there is an opportunity to reframe and humanize dying from an irredeemably grim reality to an experience that can contain richness of meaning for patients and loved ones alike. *Death Is But a Dream* illustrates an alternative sensibility and approach to care at the end, one in which the patient simply comes first.

By letting patients themselves tell us what they need and value the most, we can humanize the end-of-life process. In the words of the poet Rainer Maria Rilke, "I will not say that one should *love* death; but one should love life so magnanimously, so without calculation and selection that spontaneously one constantly includes with it and loves death too (life's averted half) . . . Only because we exclude death . . . has it turned more and more into something alien . . . something hostile."

And truly, what the dying fear most is not losing the capacity to breathe but the loss of a life they can recognize as their own, what "makes life worth living."

End-of-life experiences testify to our greatest needs—to love and be loved, to be nurtured and feel connected, to be remembered and forgiven. They provide continuity between and across lives. Based on the content of these dreams, it's obvious that the forgiveness and love that count the most come from family. As doctors, we owe it to our patients to support and facilitate their capacity for self-healing and self-nurture. Sometimes, that means standing out of the way so that people like Tom can be reunited with and comforted by long-lost mothers and so grieving mothers like Mary, to whom I will introduce you next, can once again hold their deceased children.

I am a doctor, and all my patients die. Despite the tremendous loss inherent in these words, there is light within the darkness of dying as most patients find a path to affirming the love they felt, the relationships they cherished, and the life they led. This book is their story.

# from there to here

Do not believe that he who seeks to comfort you lives
untroubled among the simple and quiet words that sometimes
do you good . . . Were it otherwise he would never have been
able to find those words.

—RAINER MARIA RILKE

The making of a doctor is a process with a beginning, middle, and no end. Student doctors leave the halls of medical school with vast amounts of information and knowledge that they will eagerly dispense to their patients. When they arrive at the hospital for the next phase of their apprenticeship, they have learned about disease and have yet to learn about illness: the former occurs in organs; the latter in people. The last and most important phase of their training will be lifelong. This is when the patient teaches them, and they are hopefully ready to listen and humble enough to hear. This is when they learn that sometimes the best way to treat a failing human heart is to set the stethoscope aside and ask about what matters to the patient, rather than just what is the matter with them. And one day, just when they think they have mastered the science of medicine, they will meet a patient who will summon them to tend to the soul. This moment will hold a lesson in empathy these doctors will never forget, the first of many through which they will find the true richness of the calling. The patient who first guided me through that moment was Mary.

Mary was a seventy-year-old artist and mother of four, and one of my first patients at Hospice Buffalo. I once visited her room when her "whole gang," as she called them, was gathered around her sharing a bottle of wine. It was a low-key family affair, with Mary appearing to enjoy the company of her brood, even as she drifted in and out of alertness. Then something odd happened. With no prompting whatsoever, Mary started to cuddle a baby only she could see. Sitting up in her hospital bed, it was as if she'd lost touch with the here and now and was acting out a scene from a play, kissing this imaginary baby in her arms, cooing to him, stroking his head, and calling him Danny. Even more striking, this incomprehensible moment of maternal connection seemed to have put her in a state of bliss. Her kids all looked at me, uttering variations of "What's happening? Is she hallucinating? This is a drug reaction, right?"

I may not have been able to explain what was happening or why, but I did understand that the only appropriate response at that moment was to refrain from intervening medically in any way. There was no pain to alleviate, no medical concern to address. What I saw was a human being experiencing an unseen yet tangible love, all beyond my medical understanding and reach.

With Tom, it was nurse Nancy who had relayed his dream experiences to me. I neither witnessed them nor could have them corroborated. By contrast, with Mary, I was observing firsthand the undeniable state of comfort and ease with which she was approaching the end of her life's journey. Refuting this was no more an option than explaining it.

I watched in awe, as did her grown children. After their initial outburst, they were overcome with emotion, no small part of which was due to their relief at seeing their mother's serenity. She did not need them to intervene, any more than she needed me to make a decision or say anything that could or would alter the course of her last moments. Mary was tapping into an inner resource none of us knew she had. The feeling of gratitude and peace that overtook us was like no other.

The next day, Mary's sister came in from out of town and unraveled the mystery. Long before any of Mary's four children came into the world, she had given birth to a stillborn baby she had named Danny. She was overcome with grief after losing the baby, but she'd never spoken of it, which is why none of her surviving offspring even knew about him. Yet in this moment, with death waiting in the wings, the experience of new life had returned to Mary in a manner that clearly provided warmth and love, and maybe even some small compensation for her loss. At death's door, she was revisiting her past trauma as a wrong redressed. She had reached a palpable level of acceptance and even looked like a younger version of herself. Mary's physical ills couldn't be cured, but it appeared that her spiritual wounds were being tended to. Not long after this remarkable episode, Mary died peacefully, but not before transforming what I understood "dying peacefully" to mean. There was something intrinsic to Mary's dying process that was not only therapeutic but that also unfolded independently of the ministrations of her caretakers, including her doctor.

⸎

The irony of caring for patients whose needs are as spiritual as they are medical was not lost on me. I went through medical school with a deep aversion to the nonphysical aspects of dying that stemmed from losing a parent in childhood.

The last time I saw my father I was twelve. I remember my mother stepping outside his hospital room to speak with my uncle, leaving me alone with my dad, as he lay there, dying. He began to fiddle with the buttons on my jacket, telling me to get ready because he was going to take me fishing at our cottage up north in Canada. I knew there was something slightly off about this plan, but I also knew that whatever he was experiencing was okay. In fact, it was very comforting to me that he seemed at peace, and that we were together, and that he wanted to take me fishing. I also intuitively knew that this was the last time I was going to see him. As I reached out to touch him, a priest came in and pulled me away. "Your father is delusional. You should go."

My dad died later that night. I was too young to find the words to express the feelings of loss that would remain with me the rest of my life.

I never mentioned let alone discussed what I'd witnessed at my father's bedside. It was only half a lifetime later, when I was preparing for my TED Talk on pre-death dreams and visions, that the irony of all this struck me. In a way, my whole life's work could be traced back to this powerful event from childhood, and I'd never connected the dots.

Like my father, I became a doctor. As strange as it may sound, if you have an aversion to death, medical school is a safe place to be: the word *death* is rarely mentioned, let alone the experiences patients have leading up to it. Medical training is about defying death, and if death can't be defied, then it is essentially denied, in whole or in part.

I first came to realize this when attending to dying patients during my pre-rounds as a resident. My job was to complete the "pre-rounding," which consisted of going from bed to bed, usually at five a.m., to collect patient information before the chief resident made the official rounds an hour later. The word *resident* could not have been better chosen. The position involved literally residing at the hospital while putting in eighty- to one-hundred-hour workweeks.

During that time, I silently and uneasily witnessed the practice of "signing off," shorthand for when doctors stop following a terminal patient. We not only abandoned critically ill patients, we did so by speaking the worst words anyone could say to someone suffering and in need: "There is nothing left that we can do." From a medical perspective, there was nothing more to be diagnosed or treated; from the point of view of a doctor in training, nothing to be learned. This process of elimination by paperwork was my first encounter with the institutional abandonment of dying patients, and it was part and parcel of my training as a doctor. I would one day come to realize that there is, in fact, a lot left that we can do: we can resurrect the lost art of bedside medicine and care for those who are dying by being present and relieving suffering—which entails more than just pain management—when a cure is not achievable.

After a residency in internal medicine, I began a fellowship in cardiology. The year was 1999, and several factors led me to start working part time at Hospice Buffalo. As a fellow I struggled to make ends meet with two children in a one-income household, so I always moonlighted to pay bills, mostly in ERs. As a result, I carried a pager at all times, so any additional position I took on would have to allow me to go back to the hospital in the event of an emergency.

One sleepless night, I set out to read the paper front to back and noticed a boxed ad in the classifieds section, a job advertisement for a doctor at Hospice Buffalo. I thought: "Who places a want ad for a doctor?" A more pertinent question, which didn't occur to me at the time, would have been "What sort of doctor answers a want ad?" I wasn't even sure what a hospice doctor really did because I had successfully petitioned to get out of the hospice rotation when I was a resident. Few medical students take courses in geriatrics or palliative medicine. They try to avoid facing death and want to pursue the profession's idealistic yearnings to cure. I was no exception. In many ways, I was completely oblivious to death despite witnessing it firsthand, often at the hospital. I knew close to nothing about what it meant to be a doctor to the dying.

Today, we live with a death-avoidance model of care that is

inadvertently reinforced by a fee-for-service health-care marketplace based on outputs rather than outcomes, volume rather than value. What dictates patient care is in part determined by billable products and services provided in the form of imaging, labs, and procedures. In such a context, it's often easier to get CAT scans than practical assistance at home. This is a symptom of the mismatch between the care that is needed and the services that are delivered. By its very design, our system is often unable to recognize dying patients who may simply need attention in the form of presence, care, and comfort, not "acts of doing" or billable interventions. This is why the modern death ritual has so many people spending their last days in emergency rooms and intensive care units—because that is where modern medicine recognizes them as patients. The "nearly dead" are sentenced to a medical assembly line of the absurd, undergoing imaging that yields unnecessary information and even receiving pacemakers for hearts that aren't allowed to stop even when the rest of the body has.

Dying in the hospital is an expensive proposition that ironically leads to neither longer nor better life. We know we have a problem on our hands when the majority of Americans claim not to want to die in an institution yet most of them do. Half of all dying patients visit an emergency room within the last month of life, even though any such medical intervention has been proven to make no difference to the course or outcome of their disease. They could have had the same level of medical care and much more comfort at home.

In my time as an intern and then as a resident, I had become increasingly discouraged by a hospital medicine that processed people like they were paper. I was certainly exposed to devoted doctors, but I was also working with many who had lost interest in patients as people; they merely completed tasks and filed forms and dictated notes. A widening bureaucratic gap was separating doctors from the bedside, so much so that many of my colleagues had stopped finding personal meaning in their work. Every hour of interaction with patients meant two hours of meetings and documentation. They were swallowed up by the economics of medicine. I never objected to the demands of being a doctor, but witnessing destroyed vocations was getting to me.

I had come to realize how right a fellow physician's assessment was when he warned, "Today, healing is replaced with treating, caring is supplanted by managing, and the art of listening is taken over by technological procedures." Dr. Bernard Lown, professor emeritus of cardiology at Harvard, wrote this more than two decades ago, and the trend toward an impersonal and technological medicine has only gotten more pronounced. Too often healing continues to be sacrificed in the name of treatment. And when treatment is no longer an option, doctors often forsake healing altogether.

I knew then that to survive and excel in medicine, I would need to experience it at a more immediate and genuine level. So, barely informed, I contacted Hospice Buffalo and inquired about an interview for a weekend job.

I was aware of the irony that getting this job would mean caring for the very patients I had "signed off" on at my other job. I wasn't exactly sure what a doctor's role at a hospice center was, so I went to the interview with some of the implicit bias against the job inculcated in me by my medical training, and thinking, "What kind of doctor works in hospice?"

At the end of what turned into a two-hour conversation, I asked my interviewer, Dr. Robert Milch, one of the founders of Hospice Buffalo, what qualities were necessary to be a good palliative care doctor, and he answered, "Righteous indignation." I had walked in ignorant and somewhat ambivalent. I left enlightened and powerfully motivated. And I never looked back.

When I told the Cardiology Department that I was leaving to pursue a career at Hospice Buffalo, I received puzzled encouragement from some and downright ridicule from others. One doctor said that hospice was something you did when you retired. Another doctor suggested I go see a psychiatrist. Most saw my career move as a waste of a professional life. It was true that those involved in Hospice Buffalo were primarily volunteers and retirees, but they were also ordinary men and women who, at bedside, became extraordinary. I watched more than one gruff and sullen senior colleague transform into the most tender and attentive caretaker when tending to dying patients. I was joining this organization at a time when I was disillusioned with the bureaucratic and impersonal nature of the medical profession, and these men and women were instrumental in helping me reconnect with a more humanist medicine. This was the kind of medicine my father had practiced.

One of my earliest and most vivid childhood recollections is of sitting impatiently in the waiting area of an emergency room, eager for my father to finish his shift so we could go to a hockey game. Sitting around the corner from the exam room, I heard part of his interaction with a sick patient. The way he was talking made me think this person must be somebody really important. I had not seen the patient enter and thought nothing of it until an elderly man left, thanking my dad for his time. The man's scraggly gray beard was held together by layers of grime, and he looked bewildered by the kindness he was receiving. As a homeless man, he never knew what would be coming around the corner, but in this crowded emergency room, his vulnerability was both shared and relative.

Illness is society's great equalizer, and on that day, I was seeing medicine for what it is: life struggling to care for itself. I was too young to comprehend the significance of this moment, yet its impact on me was undeniable. My father's gesture of caring may have been simple, but it was something in which I could believe. It helped me to understood why, for my dad, it was a genuine privilege to be a doctor. What I had witnessed was more captivating than the hockey game I was missing that night.

This was also the same type of medicine that defined the hospice care I was so eager to join.

---

The transition into my new position was not easy. I was a neophyte in a team of dedicated and longtime support staff among whom I had yet to find my role and prove my worth. Hospice was a nurse-coordinated movement—in part a rebuttal to traditional physician-led medicine, so doctors, including me, were met by palliative care nurses with some suspicion. After all, it was nurses who were at the bedside and who witnessed again and again the needless suffering that was sometimes caused by the failings of conventional medicine. It was nurses who recognized that the dying had needs that went far beyond physical concerns. It was nurses who saw that the unit of care was not just the patient but the patient in the context of his or her life and family. And ultimately it was nurses who remained at the bedside to provide compassionate care to those for whom there was "nothing left to do." When I joined the team, some nurses made it pretty clear that doctors were there to play a supporting role and that symbolism was important: no white coats allowed. Oversized egos were to be checked at the door.

But it was not just nurses who kept my ego in check.

One of my earliest hospice patients was Peter, a former university president who had been diagnosed with pancreatic cancer and had lost so much weight that his previously high blood pressure and blood sugar were now low. Because he was no longer seeking aggressive treatment for his terminal cancer, he had received little care oversight, and his medications had not been reviewed or adjusted. As a result, Peter was weakened to the point of debility and unable to stay awake to enjoy activities such as the political discussion groups he attended at the center. He was also towering at six feet two inches, which, combined with his weary-eyed expression and the effects of inadequate medication, made him look skeletal.

After simple adjustments to his medications, Peter was able to regain momentum, enjoy his intellectual gatherings, and recapture a sense of dignity and purpose. He then went on to suffer from a myriad of disease-related challenges and symptoms that were equally manageable, proving that the symptom demands of illness should require the same consideration as the disease itself. The lesson was clear: the need for responsible medical care does not stop just because cancer treatment does.

Peter was not the only patient I met for whom a terminal diagnosis had become a liability insofar as it obscured the management of other conditions that were actually treatable. It was possible for a patient to suffer and even die from a manageable condition such as a urinary tract infection or anemia when transitioning to a "comfort" model of care. The decision to pursue palliative care was tragically often interpreted as consent to do nothing.

Peter continued to enjoy a high quality of life even as his cancer-related pain required management, negating the idea that pain is merely a threshold between suffering and drug-induced oblivion. Dr. Cicely Saunders, who worked to develop hospice as a movement, said it best when she pointed out that there is no such thing as "*intractable* pain," although she "had met *intractable doctors*." Throughout Peter's illness, both patient and doctor learned that it was possible to live vibrantly in the process of dying, and that treatment and healing need not cancel each other out.

When I began to care for hospice patients in their homes, the absurdity of parsing them into diagnostic categories became even clearer. So did my understanding of the totality of their needs. Although they were going back to loved ones and familiar surroundings, the dying patients I saw often experienced being released from the hospital as abandonment. The ultramedicalization, constant monitoring, and expert disease management from which they had benefited in the hospital setting was abruptly cut short as they were handed over to their loving but confused families. Patients and their families had little notion of what was happening to them or what to expect. They felt like they were in medical purgatory, released from the curative modalities of medicine but unaware that there could be an alternative.

After abandonment, fear of the unknown is the next most common feeling among the dying and their loved ones. It is startling when patients and families come to you from hospitals where they know the price of coffee at the cafeteria or where to park, but they know nothing of when or how death is going to happen. Accurate and honest communication is often the first casualty as patients transition from aggressive treatment to comfort care at life's end, and this absence of information is a void often filled with fear and dread.

An overwhelming amount of data shows what the medical prognosis was like for these released patients: most died with pain or other debilitating symptoms that were likely manageable but had been ignored because of the person's impending death. As with Peter, the issue was rarely that the symptoms couldn't be addressed, but that there was only a poor or half-hearted attempt to do so. Patients were suffering not from treatment failure but from a failure to treat. There is a big difference. And let's not forget the loved ones, who were suddenly left alone and burdened with unfamiliar care demands, along with their fear of the unknown and indescribable grief. Who cared for and about the caregiver?

There was lots to do.

Palliative care demands a focus that is unrivaled in meaning and intensity. It is impossible to do this work without recognizing that what ultimately defines the human condition is vulnerability to circumstances, death, and each other. It requires that the caregiver be truly present rather than entangled in the kind of bureaucracy and record keeping that turned off so many of my peers in the practice of medicine. As odd as it may sound, it actually took caring for dying patients for me to learn to stop, sit, listen, and feel.

In the words of Dr. Francis Peabody, who taught at Harvard Medical School in the early twentieth century, "The secret for caring for the patient is in caring for the patient." Patients suffer in totality, not just in parts. If they do not compartmentalize between physical, emotional, psychological, and social sources of suffering—and they don't—then neither should we as their caretakers. A true holistic approach to patient care must also honor and facilitate patients' subjective experiences and allow them to transform the dying process from a story of mere physical decline to one of spiritual ascension. Like living, dying emerges from a rich inner life whose beauty and reach transcend the limitations of the body as well as those of medicine.

To be able to care for patients such as Mary as she was dreaming of her stillborn baby or Peter as he fought to reclaim his intellect, I needed to expand my understanding of what matters most to the patient—what and whom they had loved and lost. The process that brought about this awareness also forced me to recognize that what we bring to the bedside as doctors is a function not just of what we know but also of who we are, how we love, and whom we have lost. Ultimately, this awareness may prove to be most redeeming in our shared struggle to stay humane.

My father left me in pieces as a boy, but he also graced me with his magnificent example, and in his final moments, I was left with a question about the meaning of it all. This book is my attempt at providing an answer.

⁕

# stumbling out the gate

*You don't understand. It's not about what he's thinking,
it's about what he is feeling.*

—BETTY, WIFE OF A SOLDIER

I was an intern doing morning rounds when I walked into the room of a patient named Bobbie. She was a middle-aged woman of average build who could hold people's gaze so intently that they would inevitably have to lower their eyes. I liked her. She let nothing and no one intimidate her. I asked her how she was doing. She responded, "Okay, except for those damn pink spiders on the wall—do you see them?" I froze, checked the wall, looked at her, then turned again to face the wall. I hesitated, took a gamble, and replied no. She chuckled and said, "Good, I was testing you."

The next day I was doing rounds with a senior resident, and it was his turn to inquire about her health. She answered, "Okay, but I'm worried about those damn pink spiders on the wall—do you see them?" He paused, pondered for a split second, and stepped in it: "Why, yes I do." Bobbie stared him down and said, "Well, then you'd better go see a doctor quick, because you're nuts."

This memory of Bobbie's test still makes me smile. You have to admire someone who can invert the doctor-patient relationship with such a wicked sense of humor while tethered to a bed by both a catheter and an IV. At another, more serious level, however, the story also speaks to the challenge of entering unshared worlds. It helps expose the difficulty doctors face when they have to interpret the inner lives of their patients. Indeed, when that experience is invisible to us, our diagnosis is necessarily informed by our limited ability to assess the situation and by our predispositions. My colleague decided that the patient must be hallucinating and that it was important to validate that perspective. He was not wrong. Shattering the reality of someone who is experiencing hallucinations could send them into psychic turmoil and unsettle their sense of self, sometimes with dire consequences. By contrast, I decided that the patient must be messing with us, and I was not wrong, either. Bobbie was being herself—witty and confrontational, but not delusional. What ultimately mattered at that moment was not whether one interpretation was true and prevailed over the other but whether the patient felt reassured and supported by the patient-doctor relationship. Bobbie had to manufacture a lie detector test to determine who her most trustworthy patient advocate was.

The assessment of Bobbie's cognitive status is analogous to

the kind of evaluative work doctors have to do, often on the spot, when their patients share their end-of-life experiences. Both instances involve trying to understand the invisible inner life of patients. There too, the interpretation is in the eye of the beholder and depends on how often we have witnessed impending death, as well as our own level of comfort with this vantage point. To the uninitiated, end-of-life dreams are often just mistaken for confusional states, consequences of disease, or medication-induced hallucinations. This assessment invites a diagnosis, which is a medical label that does not always entail insight or understanding.

Within weeks of starting at Hospice Buffalo, I was at the library trying to locate sources on what I was witnessing. I found little of value in the medical literature to substantiate the dying patient's experience. Nancy had only gotten it partly right: I hadn't missed classes in medical school; there just hadn't been any offered on the subject of dying.

This is when I discovered that while modern medicine had been resolutely silent on the subject of dying, the humanities—the gateway to the subjective dimension of the human experience—had not stopped talking about it. I was reassured that others had chronicled end-of-life experiences, yet there was still a huge problem in the telling. These experiences seemed to function mainly as a welcome invitation, a blank canvas for observers to pick up a brush and impose their beliefs and explanations based on their particular philosophical, professional, or spiritual bent. Parapsychology (psi) investigators saw them as evidence of paranormal activity, of ghostly intrusions, or of the afterlife; Freudians interpreted them as expressions of repressed desires, and Jungians of hopeful ones; the religious-minded recognized in them proof of the existence of God. Most writers viewed such experiences as the elusive keyhole through which they could answer the biggest questions of them all: What lay deep within the soul and in the far beyond? Everyone was so perplexed by questions of etiology that few were intrigued by what end-of-life experiences meant to the dying. And if they were even remotely interested, few knew how to access that knowledge, often turning to bystanders instead for clarity.

In the past fifty years there has been a smattering of clinically based papers on the subject. Even so, such reports have been lacking, not only because of the inevitable bias of their investigators but also because of their methodologies. Their observations have been based either on single case reports or on surveys of caregivers to the dying, mainly nurses and doctors.

Anecdotal case reports cannot meet the criteria of scientific rigor required to count as evidence. And when it comes to the surveys of caretakers, how could something experienced at such a subjective level be adequately captured by third-person reporting? Imagine studying depression or pain by gauging the observer rather than the patient. It would look more like hearsay than like serious analysis. What I was unveiling in my library research was the urgency of the perspective from the bedside.

At the time, I was also working with University at Buffalo medical students, residents, and fellows who were doing clinical rotations as part of their training, and with whom I tried to share these insights about the dying patient's missing perspective. One day I was doing rounds with a bright young oncology fellow named Maya. As I tried to explain to her how my colleagues and I viewed and valued end-of-life experiences at

Hospice Buffalo, I saw she appeared disinterested. She commented that she was going to be a cancer doctor, which meant that she would work to fight death, not help transition into it. She seemed taken aback when I took it upon myself to remind her that patients do sometimes die from cancer. An uneasy silence ensued. It was going to be a long day.

Minutes later, we met our first patient, Jack, an older gentleman and World War II veteran who had been experiencing vivid dreams and visions of his combat experiences. His wife, Betty, a real character and all of four feet ten inches, was outside his door, standing guard to make sure that his state of mind would be properly understood. She wanted to protect him from any attempts at pharmacological intervention. She knew that he was dreaming, not delirious, that he was processing important emotions, and that he needed the space to do so.

Maya did what she had been trained to do, namely measure the patient's cognitive status by asking questions such as who the president was, what month it was, and so on. An exasperated Betty interjected that he hadn't known or cared who the president was for years. "Who the hell cares?" she said, to which my young colleague responded that this would allow her to understand if he was thinking clearly. Again, Betty eviscerated the dry clinical assessment with another breath of her humanity: "You don't understand. It's not about what he's thinking, it's about what he is feeling."

Jack had suffered with PTSD since the war. He'd had distressing dreams but was more recently reporting some in which he was finally able to rest in his foxhole and let others stand guard. Betty knew that he was being guided to a more peaceful end, and she was determined to preserve this sacred space for him at all costs.

As the day drew to its end, I asked Maya if she now believed end-of-life dreams and visions to be valid. She replied, "I did a search, and there is no *evidence* to support these observations." She believed that if end-of-life experiences did occur, they were due to traceable biological or chemical causes. She was unsure whether they happened because of brain malfunction or drug-induced hallucination, but there had to be an explanation outside of a mystical one. I was actually sympathetic to her in-transigence, having shared it in the past. Her reaction was also a jolting reminder that we live in a world where seeing is believing and where methodically collected data and evidence are prerequisites for any scientific mind. She was certainly correct—there were no studies in existence that would satisfy the medical standard of evidence. Most researchers had merely set out to prove the existence of life after death. There was no data-driven research that might change the way doctors think about death or attend to the dying.

This made it clear to me that if medical students and residents were to take pre-death experiences seriously, we would have to medicalize the phenomenon. And so we did. We set out to collect quantifiable data rather than anecdotal case reports. And so we did. We made sure that it came directly from the patients, not the observers. This was the gap that needed to be filled. But to reach any definitive conclusions, we also had to rule out the possibility that these experiences were just manifestations of confusional states.

Even a quick online scan of the literature on the topic will reveal how often pre-death dreams and visions get confused with altered mental states. Clinicians unfamiliar with end-of-life experiences routinely discount them as hallucinations caused by medication, fever, or delirium. In doing so, they insinuate that these experiences hold little intrinsic value. Yet the distinction between pre-death dreams or visions and altered mental states is critical. Patients with delirium, by definition, exhibit disorganized thinking and an inability to interpret their surroundings, which often results in agitation, restlessness, and fear. By contrast, end-of-life experiences typically occur in patients who have clear consciousness, heightened acuity, and awareness of their surroundings. These experiences differ most from hallucinations or delirium in the nature of the responses they evoke, including inner peace, acceptance, subjective meaning, and a sense of one's impending death. The distinction matters because an inappropriate medical intervention may impair the person's ability to experience and communicate meaning at the end of life and increase the isolation experienced by the dying.

Patients in hospice frequently experience pre-death dreams and visions at the very same time as they experience fluctuating delirious states, particularly right before death. When medical staff are informed about the difference between the two, however, distinguishing between them becomes easy. I remember Brenda, a dying patient in our unit who arrived psychologically guarded and unable to rest. She kept having hallucinations of a ferocious bear on the wall, baring its teeth and tormenting her, a delirious state indeed. The vision was so terrifying to her that she would gasp for air as soon as the threatening animal reappeared. But in sleep, Brenda also had comforting dreams of dead loved ones who came back for her, dreams that alternated with the delirium. She kept saying, "I have to go alone," an anguished outburst we did not know how to interpret. We had to administer a dose of anti-anxiety medication before Brenda could relax, just enough so she could rest but not so much that it would remove the likelihood of more comforting end-of-life experiences. Brenda needed both medication and care, and the dosage for each had to be calibrated in relation to the other as well as to each stage of the dying process. But to the uninformed, her patient profile would have exclusively summoned a diagnosis of delirium.

End-of-life experiences are not delirium, but their legitimacy is confounded by the fact that it is common for patients to experience both when immediately transitioning from life to death. Neuroscientists and physicians often interpret end-of-life processes as restricted to the last few minutes or hours of a patient's life, which is when delirious states are likely to happen. These are moments when the brain is compromised by diminished oxygen and alterations in neurochemistry. But these episodes of altered brain function, mostly restricted to the last minutes to hours of life, are not the sum total of each patient's end-of-life experiences. The point of reference is what counts.

Equipped with a new awareness concerning patient care at end of life, I designed a rough sketch for a research study on pre-death experiences. I knew that the work had to be done and that, right or wrong, it had to be done by a doctor for it to be credible. I also knew that I would need approval from the institutional review board, the university body in charge of approving research projects that involve human subjects. We had been warned that such permission would be unlikely to be granted for a study involving dying patients, whose perceived vulnerability is always at the forefront of any debate concerning their care. There is a natural tendency to try to "protect" the dying to the point of not engaging with them at all. This is tragic because for many if not most of the terminally ill, the process of dying is not only isolating, it is downright lonely. Most are left alone to stare at the ceiling. Any form of interaction is likely to be less of an imposition than a saving grace.

As expected, we hit a snag when submitting the proposal to the university's institutional review board for approval, and I was summoned to defend it. At the meeting, a number of well-intentioned researchers expressed deep concern about the potential harm that could be inflicted on dying patients by questioning them about their end-of-life experiences. I made my plea, arguing that contrary to medical opinion, dying people welcome human interaction during the last stages of their life's journey, and I explained that I had never had a dying patient who wasn't glad to have someone sit down and have a conversation with them. The panel went quiet.

Down the road from the University at Buffalo, there is a state prison where Hospice Buffalo supports a program in which inmates volunteer to be caregivers to dying fellow inmates. Here death is unscripted, less managed, and more visible as a raw human experience. This alternative version is best told in the words of one of the hospice caregiver inmates:

I signed up for the hospice caregiver program two years ago because I knew something had to change. I did not want to be the person I was on the streets. I was a person who only cared for myself. These people who trained me told me that I was expected to have compassion, empathy, and gentleness. Me? No way. Anger and retaliation were my first cousins. But slowly, I was transformed. There was one brother [a dying prisoner] who asked me to do the impossible: color. Color? I had never colored in my life. I don't like coloring. And here I was, coloring pictures of Mickey Mouse and Felix the Cat! My brother had never met his grandchildren and he wanted to send them pictures of his coloring . . . something he would have done with them if he was "on the outside." He was too weak to color, so he asked me to color for and with him. Thirty days before he died, his family, who had written him off, sent him two pictures of his grandchildren, and he stared at those pictures until the day he died.

Toward the end, the once-tough caretaker sat quietly at the bedside of his "brother" and gave him the space to simply weep. Intuitively, he understood that much of suffering, as well as its lessening, may reside deep within the inner world of the dying. These prisoners, so clearly damaged and distressed, humanized death in a way that we all need to understand. They show us that one man can bring powerful and dignified comfort to another through simple presence.

After much deliberation, the members of the institutional review board did give us the green light to proceed with the study. That was the easy part. The real challenge was going to be closing the gap between physician and patient, professor and prisoner, and perhaps demonstrating that the best way to soothe the dying may be as simple as picking up a crayon.

※

# the view from the bed

Let the young [doctor] know that they will never find a more
interesting, more instructive book than the patient himself.

—GIORGIO BAGLIVI

Frank's advanced age and frailty belied the remarkable agility
of his mind. He had been admitted with severe congestive heart
failure, but at ninety-five, he was still completely aware of his
surroundings and loved a good conversation. He had collected
encyclopedic bits of baseball lore the way others do treasured
objects, and he could talk the game like no one else. He could
recount the sport's development from the very beginning of the
professional leagues; he reminisced about players, teams, seasons, and incidents in the game's history; he remembered the
first televised Major League Baseball game in 1939 and could

name the baseball legends as well as the not so famous; he boasted of the accuracy of the stats he had developed for seasons that players had not yet played. His passion for the sport had clearly sustained him since childhood, and he still derived intense satisfaction from it.

Yet despite his recall and engagement, when Frank closed his eyes to rest, his room became crowded with dead relatives that only he could see. This was a recurring phenomenon, and one I knew better than to mistake for the manifestation of a broken mind.

I remember the day I was summoned to Frank's bedside because he was demanding medication to help him rest. That morning, he had greeted his nurse, Pam, with a roaring "Where is my damn doctor?" Frank was so agitated that before I entered his room, Pam cautioned me that he was particularly cranky that day. Frank had been a steelworker and was most comfortable bending things to his will, me included. I went in to ask how he was doing, and he shot up in bed, exclaiming, "I can't sleep. Look, Doc—it's been great to see my uncle Harry, but I wish he would shut up." Turns out, Uncle Harry had been dead for forty-six years.

During the final stages of dying, the pull to sleep is typically strong, deep, and soothing. The sporadic wakefulness that at times interrupts it looks increasingly like slumber. Sometimes this trend takes an unexpected turn. The slow drift comes to a halt as the sleep-awake state is flooded with intense and lifelike dreams and visions. The exhausted patient is not always ready for this turn, and may react to it in surprising ways. Frank certainly did.

Three days before passing, he was slipping in and out of consciousness, when he suddenly cried out, in wonder, "I am in nineteen twenty-seven! I am a boy! How did they do that?" His dreams and visions were so true to life that he was compelled to inquire about the behind-the-scenes workings of the magic trick that was creating this illusion of time travel. He did not doubt that what he had seen had taken place; instead, he assumed that trickery must have been involved to make it possible. His body was shutting down, but his mind had not yet lost its foothold in consciousness. He knew where and who he was but continued to identify what he was experiencing as an alternate reality. In truth, he had a foot in two worlds, only one of which we shared.

Over time, Frank's inner-world experiences returned him to what he treasured most in life: his wife's love. The more he dreamt of her, the more he felt her presence and the more peaceful he became. He finally requested that we discontinue treatment. His decision to decline care was medically appropriate. As is so often the case, patients recognize medical futility before their physician does and, in a sense, release the doctor from an obligation that can no longer be honored. Frank wanted to join "Ruthie in heaven." We helped him reach comfort for this much-awaited reunion, and he died with the integrity he had lived and created.

More than the stamp of approval granted by the university review board, it was meeting patients like Frank that finally convinced me that collecting evidence about end-of-life experiences was a moral imperative. The dying needed their voices heard; they needed a space to describe their inner existence and the world that often lay unseen and obscured within their failing bodies. Their experiences had to be medically legitimized. Perhaps quantifiable data would finally remove the doubt about the importance of pre-death dreams and visions as sources of comfort, meaning, and self-integration; perhaps it would provide the evidence missing from the medical literature, information that would hopefully help clinicians recognize the importance of end-of-life experiences. Medicine's technical prowess is admirable only insofar as it caters to the patient's self-worth and emotional sustenance at life's end, the reality that pre-death experiences clearly demonstrate.

The path was clear, so I sat down with Dr. Anne Banas, a University at Buffalo research fellow whose enthusiasm for the study of end-of-life experiences was immediate and unequivocal. We developed the parameters and details of my research proposal. The point was to adopt an objective approach while remaining true to the patient perspective. Indeed, with the exception of some case reports, most previous studies had focused on the observer's point of view. For instance, the first large-scale examination of the experiences of dying patients, captured in the book *At the Hour of Death: A New Look at Evidence for Life after Death* by parapsychologist researchers Karlis Osis and Erlendur Haraldsson, was exclusively based on surveys and interviews of doctors and nursing staff. Certainly, their findings were invaluable. They not only helped define end-of-life experiences in great detail but also differentiated hallucinations from pre-death dreams. But the authors' hypothesis included consideration of the afterlife and was unable to give voice to patients directly. In 2008, *The Art of Dying: A Journey to Elsewhere* by

Drs. Peter and Elizabeth Fenwick also considered an afterlife hypothesis in their investigations. They too used surveys and case analyses from the perspective of health-care workers and care providers rather than the patients themselves.

Such systematic studies of end-of-life experiences are certainly *about* the dying, but they are not necessarily *for* them. When pre-death dreams and visions are used as a lens to make sense of dying, the patients themselves often recede into the background, when their perspectives should be kept front and center in any discussion of end-of-life experiences. Our study's objective was simple: first to demonstrate that pre-death dreams and visions exist and occur routinely, and second, to address their prevalence, content, and significance from the patient's perspective.

To document end-of-life experiences as told by patients themselves, we utilized a standardized questionnaire in conjunction with more open-ended questions. The first part included unambiguous questions related to the presence or absence of end-of-life dreams and visions: whether these experiences occurred during sleep or wakefulness, whether they were comforting or discomforting, and what imagery they included. We asked every participant the same questions about dream or vision content, frequency, and degree of realism. We used a numbered scale so answers could be quantified and compared.

To be part of the study, patients had to be able to consent and understand the implications of participation, which were, as per institutional review board recommendations, detailed over many pages. The document had to be read and signed in the presence of a witness. We did not include those who displayed the slightest form of cognitive impairment such as dementia, delirium, or confusion.

Participants were interviewed almost daily until their passing. Whereas previous researchers had collected data only during random moments very near death, we examined dying as a process that lasts from days to months.

In addition to collecting data, we filmed patients. The decision to do so was meant to further corroborate and better represent the patient perspective. It also functioned as the ultimate rebuttal to the notion that end-of-life experiences are merely manifestations of a cognitively impaired or confused mind. We wanted to show that dying patients are not just what they are too often imagined to be—faded, lethargic, and often time-ravaged people in hospital gowns, too frail to function or think. Rather, they represent the full diversity of the living; they may be alert, contemplative, thoughtful, or intuitive, young or old, able-bodied or disabled. They are each unique in their own way.

It soon became apparent to every member of our team that while we may have been behind the methodical and objective approach that framed the study, we were not actually the driving force behind it; the patients were. It was those dying who propelled the research forward, in ways we sometimes had not anticipated.

For most of our study's participants, it was gratifying to be heard at all. For many, it was heartening to know that their pre-death dreams and visions warranted serious inquiry, while for others it was a chance to contribute. When a film crew approached Hospice Buffalo about producing a documentary based on the research project, every patient we consulted was on board with that too. They all appreciated being part of something meaningful that transcended their immediate preoccupation with and experience of dying. They were also no longer alone. We were always met with interest, often with relief, and at times even with gratitude. The question "You mean, you don't think I am crazy?" became a mantra of sorts. Our patients were not objects of study; they were collaborators, commentators, co-investigators, subjects, and stars, all rolled into one.

Originally, the motivation behind the study was to provide the evidence required to convince medical colleagues of the clinical relevance of end-of-life experiences. But we were holding the wrong end of the stick. As evidence-based as our study was, its findings left my fellow physicians utterly unimpressed and uninterested. More so than the medical profession, our real audience was the caretakers—the mothers and fathers, brothers and sisters, aunts and uncles, the grown children, and anyone else who has to confront the loss of a loved one; in other words, the living. And yes, that also includes doctors, but for some, maybe not until they have taken off their white coat and returned home to those they love.

Our research was for patients and families for whom end-of-life processes either triggered a fear of ridicule or a label of cognitive decline. These were the people who were the most likely to one day reach—and teach—their medical providers, just like they had taught me.

I remember Bridget, an eighty-one-year-old devoted Lutheran grandmother with chronic obstructive lung disease, who was so uneasy about the implications of her visions that she grew increasingly and uncharacteristically quiet. When her dreams became so vivid that they seemed to blend into her awake state, she repeatedly asked, "Why am I seeing this? Am I going crazy?" and her daughter, herself uncertain, did not know what to say. Bridget shared her recurring dream of two dead aunts who were standing and watching over her. These were followed by visions of her mother dressed in a long, luminous white dress and sitting at the dining room table crocheting. Although without voice, this figure was also a powerfully felt presence. Bridget could not come to terms with what she herself described as her "visions." They created somewhat of a crisis of faith, because at life's end, she could not reconcile what she saw with the precepts of her religion. She expected to see angels, not dead people.

The weight of the world was lifted off Bridget's shoulders when we explained to her how common these end-of-life visions were, that what was happening to her was no anecdotal oddity but a recognized and studied phenomenon. It helped to cite the results of our study: that the vast majority of our patients— more than 80 percent, in fact—had reported at least one end-of-life experience during their enrollment in our research. From that point on, Bridget became so comfortable discussing her end-of-life experiences that, sensing my aversion to the supernatural, she delighted in telling me that spirits like to follow the living, especially disbelieving doctors.

When patients have their pre-death dreams and visions validated, life's end can become a journey toward a transformed state, often of wholeness regained. Our study confirmed that end-of-life experiences help patients connect and reconnect to who they are and to those they loved and who loved them back. They become a way of preserving or resurrecting the integrity of the self. Within the words of our dying patients were illuminating stories of deeper meaning, an inner journey through which selves were honored, wounds were healed, and bonds were restored. For many, this meant reuniting with those who loved them best and they needed most.

Like Bridget, Ryan, a fifty-one-year-old Protestant with metastatic colorectal cancer, was initially worried: "Am I losing my mind? I haven't seen some of these people in years." But when his dreams and visions ceased in correlation with clinical improvement, he sighed, "I am back to reality. I miss the other stuff."

Ryan had never married, and never moved out of the neighborhood in which he had been raised. By any measure, he had experienced limited success in his career but found tremendous joy in life's simple pleasures and dependable affections. He had a loyal group of friends, most of whom he knew from childhood. He loved the 1970s and the music and culture that had shaped his youth, and he had shown no inclination to move beyond that decade. His point of reference had remained safely anchored in a past of rock and roll—a virtual time capsule. Now dying, he dreamed of both living and deceased friends, with whom he was going to every concert he had ever attended; he revisited the weekly garage sales through which he casually roamed, mostly looking for old record albums; he went fishing in the local river. At other times, he "traveled with relatives," although he never knew where they were going. In these moments, he felt alive amid cherished memories, unburdened by the limitations of his illness. The physical complications that came with dying had been an affront to Ryan because they had compromised his socially active lifestyle. It took reexperiencing freedom in his end-of-life dreams for him to reach acceptance. Now, despite his physical decline, he again felt the warmth of familiarity and cheerful living that had defined his existence, one rich with friends, music, and small adventures.

Our studies revealed that as patients neared death, dream content shifted from a focus on the living to a focus on the dead. The most important pattern was twofold: as people approached death, their end-of-life experiences increased in frequency, while the content of those experiences featured more deceased than living loved ones. It turns out nurse Nancy was right to scold me for my disbelief; she may indeed have been able to predict approaching death when Tom began having more dreams of his deceased mother. And although Frank remained relatively alert until the end, the increased sleep disturbance he experienced due to his multiplying dead visitors also alerted us that he was nearing the end. It appears that dreams of the deceased hold prognostic significance based on changes in frequency and content as the end draws near.

Also pertinent is the fact that end-of-life experiences involving deceased relatives and friends were shown to provide the highest comfort rating among our patients. In a startling reversal of our cultural association of death with grief, sadness, and struggle, the numbers spoke for themselves: Patients on average rated the comfort level of seeing the dead as 4.08 out of 5 (with 5 being the highest comfort), compared with an average of 2.86 out of 5 when seeing the living. And the end-of-life experiences that they most frequently reported as soothing included the presence of dead friends and relatives (72 percent) followed, in order, by living friends and relatives, dead pets or other animals, past meaningful experiences, and finally, religious figures. Taken together, the data suggests that the dying process includes an extraordinary but built-in mechanism that soothes our fears as our inner world becomes ever more populated by those we have loved and lost. Remarkably, the greatest comfort comes from our most basic and foundational needs and relationships, and from moments that capture the beautiful simplicity of everyday life.

One of Rosemary's last dreams was of a family gathering, with everyone meeting to eat, drink, and be merry. This straightforward scene of joyful family reunion also included, however, a vision of her daughter Beth getting ready for a trip. She could see Beth preparing her suitcase as the party was winding down, and family members watching her assemble her things. Specifically, Beth was packing a selection of the beautiful, flowery silk scarves she made and sold. The contrast between the joyful family reunion and the loved one's imminent departure spoke volumes about Rosemary's ambivalence regarding the end of her life's journey, which she often verbalized. She felt sustained by the warmth of the family gathering but was also visualizing the prospect of separation, albeit in a nontraumatic way. Sometimes, a simple dream narrative can and does reflect the most complex feelings, those that seek to reconcile grief with acceptance, joy with longing, and togetherness with absence.

In another study, we identified distinct thematic categories. For instance, a large group of patients described dead friends and relatives in their dreams as "waiting for them" while standing "just there," in a quiet presence that felt like the tightest embrace. This watchful silence involved no judgment, just pure love and guidance. Bridget had no doubt about the supportive nature of her vision when her two dead aunts appeared to her, simply standing and watching silently over her as she slept. She could sense the ubiquity of their love.

More than one-third of our participants identified travel or preparing to leave as a common theme in their dreams and visions. And interestingly, as with Ryan, the absence of a travel destination was typically a source of peace, not anxiety. Again and again, patients described themselves and others boarding planes and trains, riding in cars and buses, taking taxis and other modes of transportation, while identifying the experience of preparing to depart as comforting. Being bedridden did not stop Julie, a seventy-one-year-old patient with pancreatic cancer, from dreaming of travel. In fact, it is likely that her lack of mobility was precisely the catalyst for her particular dream content. She did not, any more than Ryan, know where her trips would take her, nor did she care. Thirteen days before her death, she repeatedly reported seeing her mother and her two deceased sons at her bedside, telling her they were "coming to pick her up." A week before her death, Julie, no longer able to speak or move, nonetheless attempted to get out of bed. She just knew that she had somewhere to go.

There are multiple themes and categories that are repeated across end-of-life experiences and about which we went on to publish papers. However, what patients such as Nancy and Rosemary ultimately taught us was that what "counts" ironically defies our well-meaning thematic categories, as well as simplistic or statistical measurements.

The near-universal response we received about end-of-life experiences was that they are categorically "distinct" from "normal dreams." Some of the most common statements we recorded were "I don't normally remember my dreams but these were different," "They felt more real than real," and "It was as though it actually happened." Patients emphatically maintained that their dreams were not just lifelike, they were actually lived. When asked about the degree of realism of their end-of-life experiences, most patients rated them 10 out of 10, whether they were asleep, awake, or both. What we would refer to as "dreams," because they happened during sleep, patients themselves would call "visions," as insistently as those who claimed to have seen dead people with their eyes open. In fact, in our survey of patients, 45 percent of pre-death experiences occurred during sleep, 16 percent took place during wakefulness, and more than 39 percent happened in both states. Certainly, these statistics reflect the shifting levels of alertness that define the dying process—the bouts of realistic, lucid dreaming when patients are aware that they are dreaming, as well as sleep punctuated by a degree of dream intensity that carries over into wakefulness. But in all these cases, our patients talked about their end-of-life experiences as the most awake, alert, and present they had ever felt. While this may make it more difficult for researchers to define wakefulness at end of life, the ambiguity is completely irrelevant to the dying patient, for whom the experience is as vivid, palpable, and impactful as if it had been experienced when awake, if not more so.

When ninety-one-year-old Anne was admitted to our inpatient facility with congestive heart failure, she was having such clear visions of her long-deceased sister that upon waking one day, she looked around and asked, "Where is Emily?" Emily had been dead sixteen years, but to Anne, her presence and appearances were as real as her doctor's. Anne was subsequently admitted to our inpatient unit in acute respiratory distress, where she woke up, stared up at the ceiling, and acted as if she was seeing things that were not there. At one point, she sat up in bed and stretched her arms out to the ceiling as if to embrace someone. She asked her family, "Am I going to die now?" When her condition improved, she awoke, looked around, and asked again for her dead sister, explaining that Emily had been there all along, sitting beside her on the bed. Anne also reported having frequent dreams of a more youthful Emily, going about "doing the usual things" around the house. She could describe her sister's appearance in detail: the strong, jutting chin, the dark blond hair pulled in a high loose bun, the sagging pea green cotton jersey dress whose sleeves were rolled carelessly at the elbows. Sometimes Emily put her hand over her mouth and laughed, before moving on to the next task at hand. Few words were uttered, but the dreams were heartwarming and invigorating, with Anne often envisioning herself as much younger and going for walks with her sister. She had been one of five siblings, but she was closest to Emily, who had raised her. "I am not going alone—Emily will be with me," she insisted.

Despite my inability to share in her perception, I was grateful that she was not alone, that she was comforted and at peace. The next day, Anne continued to have dreams of her sister, and two days later, after she had stabilized clinically and resumed sleeping, she was discharged home. Like most patients, the stalling of her physical decline toward death coincided with a cessation of her pre-death experiences, and like Ryan, she regretted not having visions anymore. Anne died peacefully at home about a month later, and although I was not at her bedside when she made the transition, I doubt that she went alone.

Another striking feature of end-of-life experiences is their ability to reconstruct or edit memories. Significant moments, often derived from childhood, are condensed, modified, and restructured, so patients' most pressing needs can be addressed and redressed. Tim, a seventy-three-year-old lifelong laborer with end-stage colon cancer, had end-of-life experiences that both evoked and restructured his childhood memories so he could relive them free from the pain of the poverty with which he had grown up. He first began seeing his parents, grandparents, and old friends, who kept "telling me I will be okay." Then, four days before he passed on, his dreams placed him back in the formative years of his early teens. He had grown up amid the tragedies of the Great Depression, in a blue-collar neighborhood of South Buffalo, where he had helplessly watched lives get broken and displaced. His father had fought to support his family with low-paying and sporadic work. Like many who lived through those hard times, the single most important fear that overshadowed his happiness was about the family's collective struggle to make ends meet and find hope and purpose among the despair.

Tim's end-of-life dreams helped ease the burden of insecurity this pivotal period in his life had occasioned. He reimagined himself as a young boy walking through and out of his house, a metaphor for his childhood journey. First, he passed the kitchen, where from the corner of his eye he could see his mother kneeling in prayer. The meaning was clear: Tim had described his mother's devotion to God as his family's source of strength. He then saw himself walking out of the house, only to be overtaken by his best friend, who lived next door. The boy was holding a baseball bat and a ball and summoning Tim to come and play. Significantly, this friend would remain his life-long best friend and one day even become his brother-in-law. Finally, he saw his father pushing a wheelbarrow, a sign of employment and a sense of worth restored. Tim's old psychic wounds were healed; his world was now safe, sustaining, and complete.

As Tim recounted his dream, I was no longer looking at a frail, dying man but at the sparkling eyes of a child who had rediscovered the early love that had nurtured and warmed his life. What had first looked like the separate stages of a three-act play—his mom in prayer, his friend playing ball, and his dad walking off to work—provided unified visions of the most important forces in his early life, variants on the same theme of love. These were rich and connective enactments of the layered relationships that had mattered to him most growing up and that made him who he was. They offered a multifaceted and meaningful version of an imagined but essential reality in response to his most deep-seated fears and needs. Tim himself interpreted his dream as an archetypal resolution that brought him back to a feeling of wholeness and peace. He felt a profound sense of connection that, as for many other patients, transcended words and language. In end-of-life experiences, little may be said but much is understood.

Tim's dreams condensed, reordered, and repackaged meaningful past events to put him back in touch with the most sustaining and uplifting aspects of his past life. For other patients, this reality makeover entails a much more radical editing process that excludes as much as it selects.

For eighty-nine-year-old Beverly, a patient dying of chronic obstructive lung disease, end-of-life dreams helped her reconnect with past sources of love and support by removing the person who had withheld love in the past. Beverly's childhood had been dominated by a distant and abusive mother who would force her to perform hours of pointless household chores such as scrubbing furniture with a toothbrush. At death's door, Beverly's end-of-life experiences took her back to her childhood, but it was one without the mother figure who had made her feel unwanted. In her dreams, Beverly was nine again, and interacting solely with the only source of unconditional love she had known at the time, her father. She saw herself reliving a childhood ritual that had sustained her in young life. In her dream, she was eagerly waiting for the moment after school when she could join her father on his mail delivery route. She had learned all his routes by heart and knew exactly when he'd appear by the clearing at the edge of the woods, far from their home. She would scamper to him joyfully and hold his hand as they walked the rest of his route. As Beverly neared death, the passing decades blurred to irrelevance, her negative memories vanished, and all that mattered was the warmth of her father's love, which took her from present to past and back.

We had designed the study thinking the therapeutic value of end-of-life experiences resided in easing the dying process. We had no idea that their potency extended to injuries whose genesis could be traced back to childhood. End-of-life experiences are not just about life's final transition; they address life in its entirety. Sometimes, they do so by cutting out the injurious past or by offering an alternate ending. The means are as varied as the goal is consistent, namely the resolution of what was once a crippling affliction into healing and redress.

My eighty-eight-year-old patient Scott was a case in point. He had grown up as one of eight children in an impoverished Buffalo working-class family during the Depression, a past his end-of-life experiences resurrected when it was time to revisit his life's biggest trauma. At age ten, Scott lost his right arm while jumping trains with his friends. What ensued was a childhood of teasing and a lifetime of struggle that haunted him to the end. At this tender age, he suddenly had difficulty with the most basic tasks of everyday existence such as bathing or changing clothes; he could not play with friends, who saw him as an oddity. Even his mother's love turned to palpable fear at a time when growing into a man meant finding employment for basic sustenance, and employment was limited to the whole-bodied. She had gone so far as to place him as a teenager in foster care to "get a better education," a decision that exacerbated his shame and doubt about being able to live independently or to be loved. Later, despite finding steady work in maintenance, he continued to be haunted by the impact of his childhood trauma, a victimization he could not shake. His fear had extended beyond his concerns about holding a job to his personal identity.

Shortly before his death, however, Scott began to dream of "good times at work." Now, near death, his end-of-life experiences featured him performing his job well and fixing problems that nobody else could solve. Where there was doubt before, he now excelled. Eventually, he would even dream of old colleagues taking turns to reassure him that he was "a great worker and a friend." His release from old injuries, both physical and psychic, had demanded the rewriting of past events so he could feel whole again. The irreversible wounds he had incurred both bodily and spiritually in his youth were redressed in life's final moments.

A similar process defined the end-of-life experiences of a decorated war veteran who was admitted to our facility due to persistent insomnia. John had been diagnosed with end-stage heart failure, but that was not what kept him up at night. When I walked into his room, I was struck by this broad-shouldered man who wore the distraught and exhausted face of someone who had seen too much. John had participated in the battle that General Eisenhower had named the Great Crusade of World War II, the Battle of Normandy. When I asked him about his condition, he summed it up with three words: "A war problem." He then let his family members elaborate.

John's family explained that although he had never so much as mentioned his war experiences until the previous few weeks, he was now unable to close his eyes without reliving the unimaginable carnage of D-Day. He had recurring nightmares, from which he woke up drenched in sweat. It took his end-of-life experiences for John to come to terms with the haunting memories of war. He went on to share with me details of the past he had kept from his family. Maybe he had wanted to spare his loved ones the knowledge of the agony and nightmares that had defined his troubled sleep after the war, or perhaps he could not find words to describe his horror.

John was only twenty when he enrolled as a gunner on the SS *James L. Ackerson*, which entered Normandy beside the USS *Texas*. He was and would always remain a proud Texan who took his duty as a soldier to heart and believed in the ideals of his country. On June 7, 1944, he was part of the infantry division that was sent ashore to Omaha, the bloodiest of the D-Day beaches. Their assignment was to retrieve the soldiers who had been isolated from the rest of the forces ashore. The mission was successful and the landing craft came back with the wounded Rangers they had been sent to rescue. Still, John would never be able to wipe away the vision of the bloodied beach strewn with the mutilated bodies and floating limbs he saw upon landing. This was the experience in the war that was going to haunt him for the rest of his life.

As he lay dying in hospice, John was assailed by nightmares about the fallen American soldiers he could not save: "There is nothing but death, dead soldiers all around me." I had witnessed people in a state of fear before, but John was not just frightened; he was terrified. His terror was palpable. I had never been able to adjust to the idea of a young man facing the horrors of war, the possibility of death at life's beginning, but watching John return to that site of terror a second time as an old man defied words. He described his nightmares as so intensely real that they felt lived. He could not overcome his pain, and his dreams reflected it.

This is why the complete transformation he underwent a few days later was all the more remarkable. I went to see him, and he was visibly comfortable, even at peace—he could sleep, he said, smiling. He credited two of his more recent dreams for this welcome development. In a first joyful dream, he had relived the day he had finally gotten his discharge papers from the military. His second dream sounded more like a nightmare, but to him it was anything but. He dreamt he was approached by a soldier who had been killed on Omaha Beach and had come back to tell him: "Soon, they are going to come and get you." John instinctively knew that "they" referred to his fellow soldiers, and that the dream was about reuniting with his comrades, not being judged. He finally had closure. He could close his eyes and rest.

John's end-of-life experience did not deny his reality or his war, but it did recast them in such a way as to grant him his hard-earned peace. The soul of that courageous twenty-year-old boy who had fought the ghosts of war for sixty-seven years was finally released from its injustice and from his sense of enormous obligation.

John's story exemplifies the process through which even the most difficult dreams can provide substantial psychological or spiritual benefits to the dying patient. For him, the tortured memory of the deadliest of the D-Day assaults morphed into the site of the very military camaraderie he thought he had betrayed. He needed to be released from the obligation he had been unable to fulfill and from the overwhelming shame he could not escape. Most importantly, he needed to forgive himself for his inability to save his brothers-in-arms. Thankfully, his pre-death dreams and visions allowed him to do just that.

End-of-life dreams and visions help fulfill each patient's unique needs, whether those are to be forgiven, to be loved, or to be granted peace. For some, their longing is so overwhelming that it affects not just dream content but also their external reality. We often hear of dying patients who wait for a particular anniversary, birthday, or visitor before taking their last breath. Prior to working at Hospice Buffalo, I assumed this phenomenon to be part of the lore that was passed around hospitals and whose origin may have been as nebulous as the evidence evoked to support it. Then I met Maisy, a ninety-eight-year-old matriarch who simply refused to pass before her son Ronnie made it to the hospital.

Maisy had not seen her son in eight years. This may have been due to an interpersonal conflict or just time's swift passage. There are questions better left unasked. She had stopped eating several days earlier and was no longer verbal, so we knew she was teetering at the threshold of death. Her relatives had gathered around and were talking freely—not with her, because she had seemingly lost consciousness, but certainly about her, the woman who had taken in more than a hundred foster kids in her lifetime. They didn't know that she could hear them. Someone mentioned that they'd had the police track down her biological son Ronnie in Oregon, and that he had booked a flight to Buffalo. They were now worried he would not make it in time to see her. The next day Maisy opened her eyes, sat up in bed, and cried out her husband's name. "Amos! My Amos!" she said, followed by "I can't come to you now. My son's coming." Ronnie arrived on the same day; twenty-four hours later, Maisy closed her eyes for the last time.

I could give a protracted explanation for what happened to allow Maisy to stall a process over which she seemingly had no control. It would have to do with sleep patterns and their relation to the dying process. I could explain that dying is progressive sleep, and that to sleep deeply one must be able to relax and let go. I could provide evidence about the biological processes involved in not yet dying, but that would not do justice to what I and others commonly witness. It would not even come close. Maisy's mind was unable to find peace until Ronnie arrived. In the final analysis, dying, like living, is about love that endures no matter what, and that finds a way to persist within the confines of our existence.

For some patients, the peace and understanding gained at end of life is achieved through dreams and visions that wash over them, summoning up images and emotions that soothe and appease. Others attain perspective through a more conscious process of reflection that they methodically apply to their end-of-life dreams and visions. These are patients who are keen on trying to understand the mysterious process through which death is somehow turned into a familiar, even welcome friend at life's end. This was true of Patricia, for instance, who had been so eager to help us move our research along. The conclusions we reached through the study were truly remarkable, but it took patients like her to give them a human face. Patricia had such an exceptional recall of her end-of-life dreams and visions that she became one of our richest points of access to the comforts provided by these experiences.

When she arrived, Patricia took Hospice Buffalo by storm. She was ninety years old, and nothing about her past, physical condition, or appearance could have prepared us for the engaged, alert, and witty person she revealed herself to be. She had advanced pulmonary fibrosis and often struggled to breathe at rest despite being permanently connected to a portable oxygen tank. Patricia's condition was so advanced that she could not walk across the room without experiencing severe respiratory distress, but she made up in verbal delivery what her body couldn't deliver in mobility. She spoke in as uninterrupted and fast a flow as an auctioneer. Talking to her for any length of time inevitably eclipsed her physical symptoms or the medical equipment she depended on, so much so that someone once remarked that she wore her nose tube like an accessory. She was so self-possessed that anything connected to her body, artificial or otherwise, looked like an extension of her, no different from the horn-rim glasses or the butterfly hairpins she wore. She was also intellectually vibrant and curious, and we found ourselves thinking of her more as an interlocutor than as a patient. Patricia maintained a desire to engage and express herself right up to the very end, even when her disease had progressed to the point where she longed to die.

Her mother had died of pneumonia when Patricia was nine, and at thirteen, she'd begun taking care of her father, who had been diagnosed with the same disease Patricia now had, pulmonary fibrosis. They did not have access to the social services that are now available to severely ill patients and their families, so caring for him was a full-time job. Patricia's description of this period in her life revealed how, in the post-Depression era, maturity at an early age was not the luxury it became for later generations of American teenagers: "I had to be a caretaker from the time I was very, very young. It was a difficult role to play at any stage but particularly difficult when you are thirteen. I never resented it, though, not until I came to these crazy dreams."

Patricia's "crazy dreams," as she put it, fascinated her. She wrote extensively about them in her diary and happily shared her abundant commentary with us. She was grateful to be around people who not only took them seriously but with whom she could discuss their singular nature. "It isn't the morphine, then?" she asked when we first broached the topic, relieved to know that experiences that mattered to her were not just drug-induced hallucinations. And after pleading with me not to sugarcoat what was happening to her, she added, "So there is a pattern to this thing? Being bossy and inquisitive, I am going to ask you a hard question: Is there any way of knowing where on this graph I am?" She had realized that there was a connection between dream frequency on the one hand and one's closeness to the end on the other, so there was no stopping her analytical mind from trying to identify a logic to the changing patterns of her dreams. Accustomed to managing lives from a young age, she was now working on managing her last moments, including anticipating her time of death.

She noticed that the deceased who appeared in her dreams seemed to "stay in their own categories." What she meant was that she might dream of church friends one day or of her sisters-in-law the next, but people from her different social circles never mixed. She noticed that settings did not seem important: "Sometimes I'm in my old room where I lived for sixty years. Other times, I'm in a place that I know is mine, but I'm not familiar with it. The setting doesn't seem to be important." She also quickly identified a difference between previous dreams and the ones she was now having: "When I am stressed, I dream of water engulfing me or of storms and tornadoes, but those dreams I have had for years, and they have nothing to do with this terminal business." I remember doing a double-take when she referred to her condition as a "terminal business." She told her visitors that she wanted to die, wrote poems about it, and expounded on it in our conversations: "I am ready, yes. Yes, I am dying. I hope that is what I want, because I am ready. If there was a mechanism to ensure a progression, I would do it . . . not suicide, never ever. But I would contemplate death, like some aboriginals do in South America. They can do that. They just think, 'I am done here,' and take their leave. If there were meditations or anything like that, I would like to try that." Her poem "Reflections in the Red Zone" echoes the same sentiment:

> I don't know how it works
> I wonder every day
> Will some specter come to take my hand
> And lead me on my way?
> And what about those lights they see
> Will they ever shine for me?
> I am more than ready every day

Despite a steady physical decline, Patricia had begun writing poetry and painting in the last year of her life. The more she was robbed of her physical strength, the harder she fought to find ways to express herself and create meaning. She produced a collection of landscapes she would give to friends and family. If they showed any appreciation for her art, she would even have it framed—after giving it, because she would not have presumed to burden them with a permanent wall fixture without their input. She had kept diaries all her life and remained, as she evocatively put it in one of her poems, "a scribbler, a dabbler, a mother, a wife" until the very end.

As her condition worsened, she increasingly spoke of death as deliverance, so much and so often that her grown children became uncomfortable, asking her to refrain from mentioning it in their presence. I could not blame them. Here was the mother they cherished, who was talking about her death, which was also their loss, as something to scratch off her to-do list. It felt to them like she was discussing her pre-death dreams as if she were conducting a laboratory experiment.

I knew better than to mistake this obsession with death and dying for cheap morbidity. Patricia had spent her life taking care of others. She had tended to her dying father at an age when most kids are preoccupied with fantasies about running away or stealing a smoke; she had lived through the war, the rationing system, the anxiety of not knowing whether her fiancé would survive his armed service to the country; and she had raised kids in a household where she'd had to "wear the pants." Having spent a lifetime managing others, she was now preparing for her own exit, as much for her sake as for theirs. After all, only the unexpected can be traumatizing, so preparing herself for death was one way of averting trauma, for herself as well as for her loved ones. Patricia had spent her life worrying about them, and she was not about to suddenly change course at its end. If anything, people's character traits get *more* pronounced with age. The following passage that she once read to me from her diary illustrates this best: "I am of no use to anyone now, I hate to think that. I have to get help with stuff and it will only get worse, I am sure. So that is why I am saying let's get on with it. I dearly love all the ones that are still here, but I can't do anything for any of them, and it is too bad that they have to bother about me. So this morning, I'd like to cry but I don't. I'd like to have my mother tell me it is ok. I'd like to wake up and walk up to Chuck [her husband] and take him by the hand and walk into the eternal sunset, but that is another story, another breath, another day."

Patricia was alternating between fear of the unknown and a sense of defeat, disguising both under a veneer of casualness she did not truly feel. It was a facade meant to reassure herself as well as others. After all, she was not one to draw attention to her troubles. "Everyone has problems," she would say. "I would never go down the hall and complain, because there is always someone worse off than I am."

Certainly, there were extreme episodes of breathlessness that would coincide with her feeling utterly dejected and pleading for a swift death, but until the last week of life, these pleas were more cries of exasperation than of conviction. On her deathbed, several days before the end, she admitted as much: "You try your darndest to get better because so many people depend on you, but now I am content to just leave everything. That started just recently." This was also when she somehow found the strength to remember and recite *Hamlet*'s famous soliloquy: "To die, to sleep. To sleep, perchance to dream—ay, there's the rub. For in that sleep of death what dreams may come."

Patricia had a way of making me do homework I should have attended to in college; I once again had to resort to Google to brush up on what it was that concerned Hamlet about the afterlife. I did so later that day and smiled, remembering how several weeks earlier, she had apologized for inadvertently interrupting me when I was handing out instructions to staff: "You'd better watch out or I'll be sitting in your seat soon," she said. I was going to miss her.

For Shakespeare's forlorn hero, the fact that we don't know what lies beyond "when we have shuffled off this mortal coil" is what makes us stretch out our suffering for so long. I suspect that what kept Patricia hanging on to life for as long as she did despite mounting pain and her exhortations to the contrary had everything to do with love: of family and of her research team at Hospice Buffalo. I am also grateful that her end-of-life experiences helped bring her, one of the most selfless human beings I knew, back in touch with her core self.

End-of-life experiences are about addressing patients' needs, whether it is being forgiven, guided, reassured, or simply loved. One of the most profound issues for Patricia throughout her life had been the premature death of her mother: "My mom died when I was nine, nine days before Christmas. She had pneumonia, and they couldn't do anything." As she described this tragic loss, the depth of the psychic wound it created became visible. She had a vivid recollection of the last thing she had said to her dying mother, probably one of the most innocently inappropriate statements she could have made in the face of death: "I got a hundred in arithmetic today." She explained, "Somehow, years later, this is what stuck with me. I've never forgotten it. I think I learned something with that too, that it would mean something to her. It meant a lot to me. It was the only gift I could give her, and I feel I gave her a gift. She died that night."

As she went on sharing the contents of this dream, Patricia also remarked, "Sometimes I think that my children don't know me at all." It was a fleeting and seemingly disconnected comment, one she took back right away. But I knew what she meant. As parents, we are less likely to share the perspective through which dreams sometimes turn us into kids. It is hard enough for the grown children of the dying to come to terms with the loss of their loving parent. Yet this is exactly what happens at life's end. Patricia was reliving the last thing she had said to her mother as a girl. She was nine years old again. "My mom was in bed, and she turned her head. She had one of those old-fashioned oxygen tents. She looked and she waved, and something in me knew that this was something beyond what I could do. They smiled and they told me, 'Say hello,' and my mother said, 'Hello.' I said, 'Hello.' I remember this."

Patients often describe the presence of loved ones in their dreams and visions as simply "being there," watching without speaking or interacting. Yet in the absence of words, written or spoken, they nonetheless experience a profound sense of connection and communion. None of us were surprised, however, when Patricia shared instead a dream with a full script and dialogue included. There was nothing typical about her in life, so how could there be in death? Patricia had spent all her years fine-tuning what a life worth living meant to her, anticipating the effects of her words and actions, and caring about others. And her end-of-life experiences reflected that.

After observing the soothing role of end-of-life experiences, we soon discovered that the dying patient is often graced with more than a feeling of comfort. A more recent study confirmed the role that pre-death dreams and visions play in post-traumatic growth as well, the growth an individual experiences after encountering stressful life events such as illness or trauma. In other words, there was adaptation—substantive, spiritual yet cognitively meaningful, a mechanism through which the patient emerges from the dying process with a positive psychological change. This was as true for Patricia, who experienced growth in personal strength, as it was for someone like Frank, whose growth was more spiritual in nature.

Those who are dying may be physically deteriorating at life's end, but the emotional and spiritual identity and connection they manifest in their dreams and visions remain unimpeded and omnipresent. In this sense, end-of-life experiences do not deny our finality so much as transcend the physicality of dying to create a more meaningful transition. They represent a therapeutic opportunity and a form of healing beyond cure.

On one of my last visits with Patricia I asked her, "Who would you want to see in your dreams going forward?" even though I already knew the answer. As predicted, she replied, "I'd like to see my mother because I never got to know her."

I went to see Patricia one last time before she died. She could no longer speak and looked unresponsive. I bent over and asked her in a whisper if she'd seen her mother, not truly expecting an answer. She smiled, nodded, and pointed upward.

Nothing was said and everything was understood.

# a
# last
# reprieve

You do not have to walk on your knees
For a hundred miles through the desert, repenting.

—MARY OLIVER

Nothing in this book is meant to suggest that death necessarily comes as a warm embrace, or that our dreams or visions are certain to provide a form of consolation. Pre-death dreams are not always soothing to the dying. In fact, up to 18 percent of end-of-life dreams among our study patients were distressing in nature. Those who have suffered trauma in their lives, for instance, may revisit it during their dying dreams, while others may be overcome by intense guilt.

At Hospice Buffalo, it was a patient named Eddie whose end-of-life experiences provided the most dramatic challenge to the idea that pre-death dreams are always harbingers of peace. Eddie was a sixty-nine-year-old former police officer who was suffering from advanced lung cancer. His care alternated between time spent at our facility, where he had many recurring pre-death dreams, and time spent at home. Unfortunately, because of his debilitating shortness of breath, Eddie spent most of his day confined to his recliner. He lived with Kim, his grown daughter from a second marriage, who did her best to tend to his needs but required assistance. He had lost his wife, Celine, his "beauty queen," to breast cancer four years earlier.

Oddly enough, his story with us began with the *New York Times*. Jan Hoffman, a reporter for the Science section of the newspaper, had contacted us about writing an article on the transformative power of end-of-life experiences. When she arrived at Hospice Buffalo, ready to conduct interviews, two of the patients she was slated to meet were otherwise occupied. I reached out to staff to identify other patients willing to discuss their dreams. A veteran nurse named Donna let me know about Eddie, whose end-of-life dreams were keeping him up at night. After ascertaining his interest in being part of the interview, she arranged for the reporter to meet him.

Naturally, in light of our conversations, Ms. Hoffman expected an illustration of the positive effects of pre-death dreams and visions on patients. Instead, she got Eddie.

The retired detective was a self-professed "rascal since early childhood" who "struggled with the devil all the time." By his own admission, his wayward tendencies defined all aspects of his past life and included "bad stuff" he had done as a detective, hard drinking, and marital indiscretions. The more ill he became, the more his dreams distressed him. He was made to re-live his questionable past and reprehensible deeds, and he was increasingly struggling with his conscience. He often tried to avoid sleep to be spared the fear and torment he knew would be awaiting him behind closed eyes. True to the adage that we die as we live, Eddie's dying experiences were as fraught as his life had been.

In fact, Eddie's visions were so terrifying that when he was first asked about his participation in the dream study, he had taken a pass because "no one should have to hear the horror I experience when I close my eyes." And because he found humor in every tragedy, he quickly added, "I am too busy anyway—all booked up."

Whether he was being confrontational or cracking a joke, Eddie was grappling with his own mortality. He eventually changed his mind about participating in the study, mostly be-cause of his overwhelming need to unburden himself. He was experiencing increasing distress, and talking about it helped.

On the day of the interview, the ex-detective was on a mission both to find and to tell his truth. Eddie did not hold anything back. In the words of his sister Maggie, he had, since childhood, been "honest . . . to a fault," even if "sometimes things are better left unsaid." During the interview, he did not even think of spar-ing his unsuspecting new audience, the *New York Times* re-porter, expressing himself in the raw and prickly manner in which he had always lived. Maybe Eddie felt that the *New York Times* was a worthy platform for laying bare what he referred to as his sins.

So Ms. Hoffman met a man whose recurring end-of-life

experiences were more about accumulated guilt and regret than about resolution. Eddie confessed to having been a "dirty cop." He was revisiting the ugly scenes of his previous wrongdoings: the times he had manufactured and planted evidence as a detective, beaten up suspects, or failed to protect the defenseless; or the time he had failed to intervene when he witnessed an assault. In other dreams, he got stabbed or shot or couldn't breathe. In fact, he was so anguished by what he saw in these dreams that he required medication to rest.

Eddie's torments were not limited to his time as a cop. He had struggled with a drinking problem, only shedding the habit when he was on the brink of losing everything: his job, his wife, and his sanity. He also felt tremendous guilt about his marital infidelities. He dreamed repeatedly of apologizing to his wife, Celine, but she either didn't respond to his entreaties or reminded him that he had broken her heart. He lived in dread at the thought that his "beauty queen" might not be waiting for him on the other side. Would she ever forgive him? Did she still love him? At death's door, his late wife was still the source of his deepest regret and most profound happiness.

Eddie shared that he had been haunted by recurring suicidal thoughts: "I have no plans of killing myself, yet I keep having these thoughts." The holiday season in particular was a time that brought back memories of Celine and family togetherness, and sent him into a severe depressive state. Two years before passing, he had pointed to the shotgun and canister of ammunition that lay within his reach and pleaded that the local police be called to confiscate his weapons: "Call nine one one and they'll just come and take the thing." On another occasion, his daughter had come home to find him with a gun in his mouth, ready to pull the trigger. She called for help, and Eddie had to be talked out of shooting himself. That time, he was hospitalized for threatening to act on his darkest thoughts. Eddie wanted to die, but it was not his illness that made him want to kill himself. It was "those disturbing flashbacks" about how he'd lived.

Following her interview with Eddie, a now disconcerted Ms. Hoffman came to find me in my office; she had been "Eddied," a term of endearment coined by staff to refer to our patient's unfiltered mode of delivery. She proceeded to tell me that she did not know what to do with Eddie's story or whether she could write the article at all. His confessions had not only been "disturbing" but also failed to corroborate her understanding of what she was there to cover, namely the life-affirming quality of end-of-life experiences. If anything, she insisted, his pre-death experiences seemed to aggravate, not relieve his "tortured soul." She asked me if I was aware of the discrepancy between our claims and his accounts.

The truth was that I had sent her in blind. And now it looked like Eddie was the exception that threatened to discredit the rule. We had worked so hard to educate others about the healing potential of end-of-life processes, and now that we had finally caught the attention of a major news outlet, everything was falling apart. I immediately phoned Donna, the referring nurse, to ask what she had been thinking when she recommended Eddie for the interview. She retorted without missing a beat, "You asked for a dreaming patient, not for a patient who was dreaming of rainbows and puppies. Next time you want Mary Poppins, just say so." I thanked her and hung up.

In the end, the article "A New Vision for Dreams of the Dying" appeared, with a description of both comforting and upsetting dreams. Ms. Hoffman chose not to opine on any potential contradiction between the two. When she did mention Eddie, she did so briefly and by referring to him as a "tortured soul." She focused on patients whose stories exemplified the positive effects of end-of-life dreams, people such as eighty-four-year-old Lucien Majors, who, nearing death from bladder cancer, spoke with delight of his dream of "driving down Clinton Street with my great pal, Carmen, and my three teenage sons." He had not spoken with Carmen in more than twenty years, and his sons were in their late fifties and early sixties, but dreaming about them brought him the joy and serenity that would remain his steady companions until the end.

For me, the publication of the article was a timely reminder that we needed to gain a better understanding of the role and impact of distressing dreams at life's end. Eddie's ghost lingered as I struggled to reconcile his experience with those of more typical patients. After all, our work's integrity depended on honoring the patient journey, whether it corroborated the conclusions we had drawn from our findings or not. So, three years after Eddie's death, I went back to our medical records about the patient whose pre-death experiences constituted the exception to the healing nature of end of life. The irony of a detective posthumously mobilizing us to do better detective work did not escape me.

What I discovered in those notes were new facets to the man we had known. I found out that the officer whose job had once included securing confessions had himself become a serial confessor at life's end: basic conversations about his health with the hospice team evolved into serious disclosures about his past. Eddie would tell anyone and everyone about the times he had acted immorally, even criminally, on the job. It hardly mattered if his caretakers were his doctor, nurses, chaplains, janitors, or visitors. Disregarding shame as a mere "earthly concern," he went on sharing the unacceptable while admitting to the intolerable. His life was on full display. Eddie was not just awaiting judgment; he was actively and obsessively seeking it.

Throughout this time of unburdening, Eddie ironically kept repeating his personal mantra about "leaving the past in the past. I can't change it so why dwell on it?" even as dwell was exactly what he did. Maybe this late-life self-flagellation was a kind of penance. Or maybe it was the ransom he had to pay to buy back the peace his distressing dreams were robbing him of at life's end. He looked back but also, at times, ahead. He would try to anticipate the forms of punishment he knew he would encounter in the afterlife: "I don't think God is going to condemn me to eternal damnation for drinking too much or womanizing. I mean, it's not like I killed anybody or anything like that. Heck, I was never even in a fistfight. He'll probably send me to purgatory for a while, though." The more his body failed, the more he felt a need to repair his soul. Time was running out, so he spoke with urgency. He struggled to reconcile the discordant aspects of his identity. He was a man who had fought for law and order but also one who had been capable of unconscionable behavior.

Mirroring his self-disclosures, Eddie's end-of-life experiences were about the considerable history of abuse, given as well as received. They took him back to the incidents of sexual molestation he had experienced as a teenager at the hands of his father's brother. Eddie had never come to terms with the effects of this trauma. He kept blaming himself for what had happened because he "benefited" from the abuse: "He would let me use his car, buy me clothes, or give me money." Robbed of his power of self-determination at the onset of adulthood, he was now doing what many victims do, reclaiming his power by ascribing responsibility to his victimized young self. After all, self-blame presumes a self is there to blame, so, by implication, it helps restore the sense of personhood that the abuse has eroded, if not shattered. For the younger Eddie, self-blame had also been the only available option, since disclosure was out of the question: "I would not have been able to tell my father; he wouldn't believe me."

Eddie, the immoral cop and tortured soul, was also a harmed little boy. We kept discovering new truths about the man. And we were not done. There was still more to uncover about him.

Years passed before I could meet with Eddie's surviving family members in hopes of gathering more information about his end-of-life experiences, this time from the perspective of the bereaved. Two of Eddie's four children, Kim and Ryan, had graciously agreed to meet to talk about their late father. Ryan was in his forties with two kids of his own, while Kim, now thirty, was devoting herself to a career in music. Kim was the daughter who had been living with Eddie at the time of his death.

Meeting with Kim and Ryan made me realize that I had not yet unearthed the full story behind Eddie's end-of-life experiences or fully comprehended their workings. The man whose distressing dreams had once confounded us had been dead for years, but he was still throwing us for a loop.

Ryan and Kim had both read the *New York Times* article and were there partly to set the record straight. Kim, in particular, explained that she had balked at the description of her dad as a "tortured soul." Yes, he had regrets, she said with emotion, but that was because he had a conscience, a traumatic past, and a life cut short by a debilitating disease. With tears in her eyes, she proceeded to defend her dad's memory. She did so movingly and eloquently, embracing his full humanity, the sinner and his sins, the charming quipster and the depressed patient, and most importantly, the love that overcame it all. She described a man of his time, for whom honor meant reluctantly retiring at fifty-one because he felt that his lung condition would impair his ability to do his job well. What if, he reasoned, shortness of breath overcame him while climbing a flight of stairs to provide backup? What if something bad happened to his partner because Eddie chose to be in denial about his illness? He would never forgive himself. So he retired. But he never really left the force, at least not mentally. Kim reminisced about how fifteen years after his last day on the job, her father was still in touch with his old unit members and attending retirement parties. Yes, Eddie had flaws and a spotty past, but he was also a great father, a much-loved police detective, and a human being who had erred, hurt, loved, repented, and paid for his sins.

I was finally meeting the loving Eddie who, according to his relatives, would "give you the shirt off his back"; Eddie the "greatest dad" to whose vigilant and uncompromising support his daughter attributed her happy childhood; and last but not least, Eddie the cherished younger brother raised by his sister Maggie, who had watched over him lovingly at the end. And maybe it was his innate charm, or the openness with which he carried the burden of his guilt, but there was also the Eddie who had endeared himself to the hospice staff, some of whom, like Donna, still remember him fondly as the humorous and insatiable conversationalist who liked to boast that he had "graduated" from Hospice Buffalo when he was discharged.

Eddie was both a flawed human being who at times had acted reprehensibly, even criminally, but also someone who had generated profound depths of love, loyalty, and understanding. And interestingly, the incongruities and contradictions that defined him would all come to be reflected in his end-of-life experiences.

Shortly before his passing, Eddie slept soundly for a straight thirty-six hours, awakening refreshed as well as inexplicably euphoric. A series of phone calls to his close relatives ensued. He contacted his two sons to let them know he loved them and was proud of their accomplishments. He phoned Maggie, who was on her way to a wake, and proceeded to inform her that she would soon be going to another—his. "I made everything right with the Lord," he added. He had arranged for a sacramental confession with his former priest Father Gallagher, telling Maggie, "I know how important it is to you, so I wanted you to know." I could not help but wonder whether that confession was truly a sign of renewed faith or whether he was just trying to please his sister, because Eddie could also be that person.

Kim remembered being dumbfounded by her father's bout

of lucidity as well as his pivot toward religion. It had come on the heels of a sharp decline in his cognitive and breathing abilities that had left him incoherent before falling asleep. In fact, she could not fathom how he had located, let alone dialed, the phone that helped him reconnect with family members. She wished she had known then what she knew now about end of life, she said, because she would have seen his temporary clarity for what it was: a last reprieve rather than a sign of clinical improvement or of death's postponement.

A few hours later, Eddie turned to Kim, smiled, and said simply, "I am going to see your mom." He then drifted to his death, quietly, at the sound of the words his daughter knew he needed to hear: "She is waiting for you, Dad."

The patient we had thought of as the poster child for distressing visions had experienced an untroubled transition after all. He had achieved solace despite all the trauma and escalating psychological turmoil that had unsettled his life and his dreams. His final journey was less of an exception than a variation on a theme. There was in his story a progression I had completely missed but that was throwing new light on our understanding of end-of-life experiences.

Eddie, the man who had been so anxious about how his sins would affect his status in the afterlife, was suddenly, near death, prioritizing the needs of others over his own. Dying had demanded his complete honesty, the kind of genuine concern and reckoning he had previously shunned. Instead of fretting over the potential of hell, he was reaching out and wishing his loved ones well. He was walking backward to his grave, but he was doing so after embracing a truth that included pain, regret, meaning, and, in keeping with his Catholic faith, repentance. Most importantly, he was emerging from the experience a better man.

All the power and wonder of medicine could not have taken a patient like Eddie from malignant despair to euphoric serenity the way his inner life did, hours before his death. There are no antidepressants or talk therapies that can match the astonishing capacity of the human soul to heal itself and find meaning, forgiveness, and peace at life's end. It may be tempting to try to determine whether it is prayer, meditation, a dream, or a nightmare that kicks dying patients into a higher level of consciousness. But what matters more than the source of this transformation is its near-miraculous and magical impact at life's end.

It is not what happens, or how, but *that* it happens that is remarkable. Dying is a process from which it is not necessary to excavate meaning if patients themselves do not make it available. There is no need to look for answers, mostly because what happens at life's end does not involve a question. It is itself the answer—a self-sustaining, inspiring, and meaningful answer that requires neither intervention nor conjecture, just presence. What unravels at end of life is a process that happens again and again, regardless of the cultural, racial, sexual, educational, national, economic, or spiritual backgrounds that seem to separate the dying. It is a universal phenomenon. And it is always about love.

We will never know what happened in the quiet recesses of Eddie's mind during the thirty-six hours before his death, what made that sleep different from the night of horror from which he awoke wanting to take his own life. Did he talk to his deceased loved ones, his own "better angels," or maybe God himself? Was he forgiven? Did he feel loved? We can only speculate. We can't even be sure that he had any dreams at all. We are, however, certain that what happened occurred when his eyes were closed and his language had turned inward. He no longer needed to tell and retell his story, to explain, justify, confess, repent, or anticipate otherworldly punishments. He no longer needed to call for attention or judgment. But it was in these inaccessible moments, when he was physically nearest death, that Eddie's inner world experienced a radical shift, one that allowed him to live his last hours aligned with his higher self.

Eddie's final thirty-six hours were transformative, but that should not obscure the fact that they followed months of reckoning as well as a lifetime of inner conflict. We had all been witness to Eddie's outward suffering. The profound humanity that lay buried beneath required moving back through time, not just by singling out a final moment. It took the vantage point of a life in its entirety, through his eyes as well as those of his family, to make sense of the full impact of his end-of-life experiences.

What Eddie's story made visible was that end-of-life experiences are never singular events. They cannot be viewed in a snapshot any more than from an outsider's perspective; they require the widest of lenses. They are circuitous, enmeshed, relational, protracted, and at times inaccessible processes through which peace is achieved, whether it is through dreams that are positively or negatively inflected. His sinuous path may have involved turns through distress and others through comfort, but it had direction and destination all the same. There are no simple answers for someone like Eddie, whose life defied our understanding of good and evil, but there is a meaningful path all the same.

In our naivete, our original study had created a binary model that viewed discomforting and comforting dreams as categorically distinct. But of course, true to life, end-of-life experiences are full of incongruous tones and textures. Thanks to patients like Eddie, we realized that having distressing dreams at life's end does not necessarily result in a disruptive or fraught dying process. Under the surface, such dreams often contain the greatest opportunity for discovery of meaning, forgiveness, and peace. They may be opposed in content but not outcome.

It was not long before echoes and patterns of Eddie's bumpy but redemptive final journey became visible in other patients' end-of-life experiences. And ironically, it was the story of a lifelong criminal and drug addict that most closely resembled the police detective's arduous evolution from guilt to solace.

In many ways, Dwayne was Eddie's alter ego: a forty-eight-year-old patient who was dying of throat cancer after a lifetime of substance abuse. He had a long history of larceny, criminal activity, and incarceration. The parallel experiences between the outlaw and the detective at end of life were striking. I believe Eddie himself would probably have found humor in a story that brings together cop and criminal.

Just like Eddie, the Dwayne we admitted to the hospice inpatient unit was a puzzle: charming, funny, sociable, warm, and completely unfazed by the life of delinquency and crime from which his disease provided a reprieve. He had lived "ripping and running," as he put it, but his demeanor, ironically, was that of a person with a clear conscience. He was not known as a violent man, even though he had killed two men in self-defense. And although the courts acquitted him on both crimes, it was hard to reconcile his past deeds with the casual nonchalance that was now his trademark. He acted as if his actions did not define who he was.

Despite his weakened bodily condition, he would try to stand up for a handshake whenever we entered his room. He jigged and jogged when he shuffled across the hallway floors, even as he had to lean on his medical walker for support. He would say things like "Everything is gonna be okay, man; God loves you" or "We are on a roll, man; we can go to the mountain." And with his inimitable cheerful and beaming smile, he would add, "But I may need another cold one."

It did not take long for me to understand that his casual manner was actually a survival mechanism. If Dwayne was carefree and seemed to float on clouds made of jokes and funny asides, it was not because he didn't care; he did not have that luxury. He had spent a lifetime living on the street and relying on hard drugs to counter the stress, fear, and pain that went hand in hand with it. His life had been about drug addiction since he was sixteen years old. The only thing that mattered was scoring the next hit and avoiding feeling sick and agitated when the effects wore off.

It had been so long since Dwayne had first turned to drugs to cope with an existence made of hardship and violence that he could not pinpoint the precise moment when addiction took over. Like most addicts, he could not explain how or when taking drugs had turned into a means of avoiding the physical and mental torture caused by their absence. He was caught in a steal-deal-use loop, in which there was no time to think or feel. Stuck in survival mode, he could not afford to stop and take notice of the suffering and harm he caused others, or himself for that matter.

For Dwayne, the drug detoxification that came from being physically confined with terminal illness did not change his outlook on life. His survival instincts remained in high gear, all the more so because he was terrified at the prospect of being sent back to the street.

"The street" was still the ominous entity Dwayne talked about with apprehension. As I listened to him describe it, I could not help but think how distant his experience was from mine. For me, the street was merely a place to go from here to there, nothing other than a means to an end. But for Dwayne, the street was home. It was where he lived but could never take anything for granted or feel safe. He didn't own the street; he was owned by it. It was not "*my* street"; it was always "*the* street," a place overrun with malevolent and violent people, constant threats, injustice, crime, fear, and pure terror. It is where he stole to secure his lifelong crack and heroin habit, where he feared for his life, and where he had killed twice in order to survive.

The Dwayne who arrived at Hospice Buffalo could not look back. Resurrecting the past was too risky an endeavor for a man who had finally reached a place of safety and physical comfort. It would have meant processing the irreconcilable, the abandonment, hunger, injustice, and the murders. In avoiding his demons, Dwayne was experiencing end of life much as he had lived.

Like Eddie, Dwayne wanted immunity from the past. His priority was guarding himself from the shame and guilt that overcame him when he glanced back at his failures and crimes. Also as with Eddie, it was ultimately his distressing end-of-life experiences that would bring him the awakening he needed, albeit just under the wire.

In his most troubled dreams, Dwayne was grabbed and stabbed at the site of his cancer: "It was this nightmare. It was like I was fighting somebody. I probably done something wrong to somebody on the street in the past, and now they caught up with me, and now they know my symptoms. It was like they were jigging the knife, trying to cut off my neck where the cancer was at. That is how I was feeling. It stopped but I still couldn't let my shoulders down; I was in pain." Dwayne experienced this violent dream as an avenging attempt on his life.

When he told the attending nurse about his stabbing nightmare, she reassured him that this was probably nothing, that "a lot of people talk in their sleep." But Dwayne would not have any of it. "No, this was real," he insisted. The nurse inquired if he needed some medication, and he nodded, "because this nightmare I just had was hurting my neck anyway." His description of the real-life effects of a wound that was inflicted in a dream state was a heartrending illustration of the concept of "total pain" described by hospice pioneer Dr. Cicely Saunders as one that includes not just psychological or emotional turmoil but also physical pain. End-of-life experiences strike such a chord in the patient near death that the very line between bodily reality and the dreamworld becomes blurred in the process.

Just as with Eddie, Dwayne's recurring dreams and visions

led to a radical shift in his demeanor and attitude at life's end. This became clearer when Dwayne was filmed for the documentary on end-of-life experiences. He was on camera and just about to tell us about his recurring dream when the man whose sashaying and quipping was legendary at Hospice Buffalo started sobbing uncontrollably. Nothing used to faze the Dwayne we knew—everything was cause for laughter—but here he was, an unrecognizably vulnerable soul who was crying his heart out, trembling and shaking, while talking in an unbroken stream of tears and words we could neither interrupt nor bear to hear. Where Eddie had shocked us because of his dream content, it was the distress with which Dwayne was sharing his end-of-life experience that was overwhelming.

Dwayne was finally allowing himself to confront rather than evade. He was now a soul in search of redemption, talking about his cancer as karma and regretting his life of "ripping and running": "One thing I do know is I hurt a lot of people and I feel bad about doing it, you know, very bad, and I just hope and pray that they do forgive me because they see what influence I was under at the time when I was trying to scheme and scam and be sick with them. I just don't want them to take that to their grave and be like 'This asshole,' excuse my French. 'Now he is messed up and he think we forgot but let's show him now what can happen.' I am not gonna lie to you, I have used drugs in my past, that is not a good thing, man, that is not a good thing. I don't want to go back to that lifestyle. It is not good for you, it is not good for me, it might be good for someone else but not for Mr. Johnson because I know where it takes me to. And I just pray to my higher power that he keeps me away from it with the help of my peers, hospice, you know, I am not really gonna say friends in the street. I had no friends because ninety-five to ninety-eight percent of my friends were doing the same thing I was doing."

Dwayne was convinced that he was facing his day of reckoning. He went on to have variations of his recurring dream, recounting that "the guy was pouring acid down my neck, burning a hole in my neck. I felt like it was coming down on me. I could picture this person who was sick. I am trying to fight off this guy from hurting me, trying to cause more pain. It is because my past is coming back at me from doing wrong. Because I am not gonna say I am a perfect guy when out there because I was ripping and running the street doing wrong to individuals I should not have." There was no doubt in Dwayne's mind that his end-of-life experiences were making him pay for his past mistakes and misdeeds, and pay he was willing to do, provided he could make amends to the person he cared most about, his daughter Brittany.

Dwayne had been given about two weeks to live, and his last wish was to be reunited with his daughter. He would not stop asking for her; he needed her forgiveness and grew increasingly restless when he found out that she was in prison. The incidence of drug abuse among children of drug addicts is disproportionately high, and his daughter had not escaped the trend. The thought of not being able to see his child threw Dwayne into severe depression.

Dwayne's doctor, Megan Farrell, petitioned to get Brittany out of prison so the father and daughter could spend his last days together, and the request was thankfully granted. We decided to keep Dwayne in the dark about our plans in case something went wrong. Brittany was released with an ankle monitor and arrived unannounced. Dwayne had already set out on his slow but steady daily walk around the facility. He was shuffling along, bent slightly forward over the frame of his walker, aided by his nurse and looking dejected, when his daughter arrived. All Brittany had to say was "Hey, old man."

Dwayne instantly froze, looked up, and straightened his shoulders. He had recognized his daughter's voice and brightened up with his biggest smile. He turned around, moved his walker to the side, snatched his arm away from the nurse, and walked over to his child with his arms outstretched, glowing with happiness. It was like a sublime electrical charge had suddenly rushed through his body, mobilizing him with renewed strength and energy. Father and daughter hugged and cried, holding on to each other for longer than they ever had. They were talking and laughing through their tears. And there wasn't a dry eye in the house.

Dwayne apologized to his daughter again and again. Pouring out of him were years of unacknowledged guilt he had suppressed to survive. He was driven to confront his past and make amends: "I did, I did take your stuff. I didn't mean to hurt you," he kept telling the daughter from whom he had stolen so much, even food stamps, to buy drugs.

Brittany's response would have melted the hardest of hearts: "I don't even care about that; I just want you to get better. It's all material stuff; it is nothing I can't get back. I can't get you back. You are the reason I am out, all because of you."

For the next four weeks—because of course Dwayne hustled death into giving him two more weeks than the initial prognosis—Brittany visited him daily, for hours on end, bringing him balloons, decorating his room, and taking pictures. They would go over the details of the day, enjoy the moment, joke about the past, and play. And for the next four weeks, Dwayne made amends for his past wrongdoings while expressing gratitude for his present blessings: "Coming here to hospice has taught me a hell of a lot; it has taught me to treat people the way you wanna be treated. I am old enough and should have known all that. I was in a closet so dark that I didn't care about the next person, I just cared about Dwayne Johnson and what Dwayne Johnson wanted, and it is not about that today in this world. That is not what it is about. It is not just me. I know deep down inside I do have a heart. I just had to bring that out of me, the good side that I know I have. I had to bring it out of me. If I don't bring that out of me, if I keep hiding it, I am not going to grow. I am going to still be stuck in one spot; I am going to stay in one spot thinking I am moving forward when I am not really going nowhere. So it taught me a great deal about how I want my life to be, how I want things to flip for the good and myself, you know. I want to do everything in my power to change my lifestyle. That is all I wanna do and be seen like I am still Dwayne but on a different page. Yes, on a different page." Dwayne had only weeks to live, and he knew it, yet he could find it in himself to talk about growth so close to the end. To say that we were humbled would not even begin to describe the effect that his words and humanity laid bare had on every single one of us.

For Dwayne, meeting his daughter was the culmination of a long process of atonement, one that his end-of-life experiences had initiated. For Brittany, who knew nothing about his distressing dreams, it meant recovering the best of a father she had loved despite all his foibles. She could tell that he was "more hurt by what he felt he had done to me than his disease." This reunion was also what would lead her to make a change in her own life. It marked the day she decided to forgo substance abuse.

For Dwayne, reuniting with his daughter gave him the meaning, protection, and mercy his own mother had denied him. Joanne, still an addict at seventy-two, had stolen her son's pain meds for her own recreational use when his illness was so advanced that he was bedridden. The person who should have loved him the most was the one who was causing his suffering, just as he had done with his own daughter, from whom he had stolen. This unnatural cycle was finally broken when he cried for forgiveness and received it. His child was loving him back and saw him as bigger than the sum of his mistakes.

Redemption is more than a notion or an idea; it is also an act. Dwayne's transformation may have been triggered by his end-of-life experiences, but it was through Brittany that salvation became actualized. It wasn't just God's forgiveness he needed, it was his child's. She became the medium through which he achieved peace and resolution. She provided a sense of safety when he was the most confused, scared, and in pain. Without her, his end-of-life experiences would not have translated into love manifest; without her, he would have had a solitary death.

Like Eddie, Dwayne needed his daughter to show him mercy before he could let go. That too may be part of the circle of life—it is the people we bring into the world who often help us leave it.

By the time he left us, Dwayne had developed quite a fan club at Hospice Buffalo. Dr. Farrell, who was well aware that his mother, his caretaker, could not be trusted with his meds, had made arrangements to keep him in our facility till the end. She also footed the bill. Like most of the staff, Dr. Farrell did not just care for Dwayne; she cared about him.

I later learned that another Buffalo clinic on whose services Dwayne had relied, the Friends of Night People, a charitable organization that helps the poor, homeless, and destitute, has Dwayne's framed picture hanging in its entrance. I was not surprised. Dwayne Earl Johnson left his mark wherever he went. Dr. Farrell put it best when she described him as "an amazing person . . . unique and impactful. Who would have ever thought that a man of his background and circumstance would have made all of us stand in our own circles wondering about him and how he influenced the world in which he lived and we lived? Two worlds so separate but so wanting to be intertwined."

Dying may truly be best defined as a time when worlds that were once separate come together. Dwayne may have lived the existence of a drug addict, but he died a man of conscience, as well as, to echo Dr. Farrell, a man of influence. The street hustler who had never received a bill in his name, had no home, car, or even a license, the man who had lost everything, died having it all. He passed away restored to his best self, a beloved father and admired human being, because as his daughter insightfully stated, "Drugs may have made him do bad things, but they never changed who he was."

End of life is often a time when good and evil are exposed and blurred as life focuses narrowly toward its finality. Judgment fades as we recognize humanity in all its magnificent forms and contradictions. As organs fail and life closes, we are left to see the person whole again, in plain view.

Both Eddie and Dwayne, cop and criminal, had distressing end-of-life experiences that led them to their day of reckoning. It is from a privileged view at the bedside that I got to see between their worlds and to identify their—and our—common humanity.

—✳—

# we die
# as
# we live

There is a land of the living and a land of the dead and the
bridge is love, the only survival, the only meaning.

—THORNTON WILDER,
*THE BRIDGE OF SAN LUIS REY*

Our patients demonstrate again and again what the dying process is truly about—the resurrection of our deepest bonds and
the reaffirmation of love, both given and received. Through their
end-of-life experiences, those dying often reestablish ties with
those who mattered most to them. In these moments, even patients with fragmented and broken lives find their way to connection and belonging.

This is why I was astounded to meet Doris, an eighty-three-
year-old patient who, after a full life with seven siblings, three
marriages, and six children, had recurring end-of-life experi-

ences that were remarkably impersonal. Yet again, here was a patient whose story didn't seem to fit. Our initial categorization of end-of-life experiences as comforting or not had failed to account for the full complexity we were witnessing. I was becoming increasingly aware that understanding patients such as Eddie, Dwayne, and Doris meant more than documenting their medical histories or providing a theory that would explicate the workings of end-of-life experiences once and for all. It required hearing their stories.

So yes, most of our patients' pre-death dreams and visions staged meaningful reunions with deceased loved ones. Doris, however, seemed to be experiencing freedom from those bonds. She had dreams of flying through the air, above crowds and buildings, unimpeded and free from fear. This was one of the most exhilarating feelings she had ever experienced. It made her feel so empowered that it conjured up images of superhero-like power: "I am flying—I can just push my feet and take off—so I said to everyone around me, 'All you have to do is have faith the size of a mustard seed and you can go too.' But I was the only person in the world who could fly around. On top of mountains, anywhere, looking down at all these people in those buildings." Doris dreamt of being weightless among undifferentiated crowds, and she found this state so joyful, she "didn't want to wake up from that one." The dream concluded with her witnessing a winged angel flying through a church's stained-glass window, to the amazement of the crowd of onlookers.

As if the impersonal quality of her dream was not surprising enough, Doris also looked me straight in the eye and claimed not to know what it was like to feel love. The feeling was not just foreign to her; it did not resonate at all. She had never felt love and had no qualms saying it again and again, as if it were the most natural thing in the world: "Love, I have a problem with that. I do what I have to do; I can say the words but I don't feel them. I watch it on TV all the time and I am thinking, 'How does that happen? Why do they close their eyes when they kiss?' Maybe it was not meant for me. I find myself asking what it is that makes these people fall in love." I was there to talk about her dreams, but their content and her statements about love, or rather lack thereof, stopped me in my tracks. It occurred to me that this is how Jan Hoffman, the *New York Times* reporter, must have felt when she interviewed Eddie. She had expected a patient who would illuminate the life-affirming quality of predeath dreams, and he had shared tales of moral depravity. I had expected a nurturing grandmother and got a flamboyant maverick who claimed not to feel love. She was fascinating and absolutely atypical. Patients have a way of keeping us on our toes.

Doris's somewhat abrupt manner of speech was something I had rarely encountered in people of her generation. I was used to the subtle, reserved, even evasive ways in which the elderly often express themselves, mostly out of consideration for others. Not so with Doris. She went straight to the point—*her* point, that is—and told it like it was. If in Winston Churchill's words, tact is "the ability to tell someone to go to hell in such a way that they look forward to the trip," Doris was graced with the aptitude for telling people to go there whether they looked forward to it or not. She used no velvet glove. I remember telling her about the study we were conducting on patients' dreams and being greeted with "What kind of doctor does that make you? What do my dreams have to do with my breathing?" I smiled. I knew it would take a book to explain.

She reminded me of Patricia. She was just as articulate and straightforward, and so spunky and upbeat that it was easy to forget about her physical frailty. She had a lung disease that produced the same debilitating bout of oxygen deprivation at the slightest physical exertion. But the similarities ended there. Indeed, where Patricia checked herself if she sensed that her words could shock or offend, Doris remained uninhibited. Her candid delivery would have sounded harsh had she not been so genuine and witty about it.

I remember how, without prompting, Doris began recounting the details of her extraordinary life. I soon came to realize that her end-of-life experiences might have been unusual in terms of content but that they aligned perfectly with how she had lived.

Her story was so out of the ordinary that parts of it had been documented in *The State Boys Rebellion*, by Pulitzer Prize–winning author Michael D'Antonio. The book used her life as an example of the beliefs of an era, describing at length how Doris's journey intersected with the shocking adoption of the tenets of American eugenics by state schools. Eugenics is the so-called science of improving a human population through controlled breeding and the engineering of desirable heritable characteristics. In the mid-twentieth century, Doris had been forced into one of the American state schools that confined children in the name of biological perfection.

Here I was, startled again as I listened to Doris casually describe events in her childhood that intersected with a shameful landmark episode of our nation's history. This is how I finally came to understand my puzzling patient and could appreciate the tragic circumstances that would lead a human being to forsake love. For Doris, love was not just a feeling that she could not process, it had also functioned as a real liability in her struggle for survival.

Doris had grown up in Newburyport, Massachusetts, as one of eight poor children. Her father, Thomas, was an amateur boxer who had a criminal record that was as long as his drinking problem was deep. He was abusive, especially to her mother, Ruth, a self-effacing woman whom Doris described as "too afraid to fight back." Doris remembered waking in the middle of the night to the sounds of their dad beating and raping their mom: "We were not sure what was happening, but we knew that he was hurting her and that she hated it." Doris kept quiet in the dark, waiting for the violence to end while holding her siblings tight. Lice and fleas had the run of the single bed she shared with her brothers. They lived in complete "squalor," with filth, rats, and even human excrement that sometimes littered the floor for days. From the outside, the wooden house looked abandoned.

Doris vividly remembered the day they were intercepted by state authorities while trying to collect coal from a company yard. Ruth had directed them to crawl under the fence to retrieve lumps to heat their home. They were all arrested, and Doris would long remember her mom's traumatized stare when court officials admonished the dejected woman for being "slovenly" and "lazy" and failing to properly care for her children. The tears were streaming down Ruth's cheeks, and Doris could still see the deep tracks they had carved in the crusted dirt that covered her mother's face. This may be why the daughter would go on condemning not the mother who could not protect her but love itself, this thing she saw praised ad infinitum in human relationships, on TV, and in movies, but that could not keep her safe.

Days later, state social workers appeared at their house in her parents' absence. With the promise of free ice-cream cones, they coaxed the children away. Doris was subsequently taken to one foster home, while two of her brothers, Albert and Robert, were escorted to another. She was eight years old. She would never again see her mother, and it would take years before she could reunite with these two brothers, the only siblings with whom she had reconnected.

Motherly love may have been the first to fail Doris, but the foster homes where the state placed Doris and her brothers were no safer than the home from which they had been taken. Doris and her siblings were subjected to years of abuse and neglect at the hands of complete strangers. They were eventually transferred to the Walter E. Fernald State School, the institution where she would spend four of her most formative years, from ages twelve to sixteen. This is also the state school that D'Antonio's *The State Boys Rebellion* singles out in discussing the horrors of American eugenics, and to which I turned to find clues about Doris's perplexing end-of-life experiences.

I discovered that Fernald, as it came to be known, had been founded in 1848 to help those deemed untrainable learn skills needed for life on their own. But by the time Doris and her brothers arrived there in the 1940s, the school had long left its philanthropic mission behind to embrace the goals and aspirations of the eugenics movement. This was a time when those considered weak of intellect were no longer seen as a test of our humanity but as a threat to it. Pseudoscientists had transposed the principles of selective breeding from animal husbandry to human beings, so that testing for deficient genes had become a way to divide humans into the worthy and the others. Intelligence was seen as inherited and as fixed as eye color. In fact, words such as *moron*, *idiot*, and *imbecile* were used as medical terms.

It was shocking to read about this chapter of American history, when experts chose to ignore the overwhelming evidence that showed the role a chaotic environment and lack of education played in children's development. That was the case for Doris and her siblings, whose family life had been beset with alcoholism, domestic violence, unemployment, and poverty. She and her siblings were simply deemed "retarded."

Being institutionalized in a school like Fernald meant that Doris was surrounded by authority figures who did not believe that she could improve, let alone be trained, reformed, and reintegrated into society. Upon arrival at Fernald, Doris was tested for mental deficiency, the result being a foregone conclusion for kids from her background. She vividly described how for her twelve-year-old self, being evaluated by a psychologist, "a woman who came in with this cane, dragging her leg," was a terrifying experience. She remembered shaking uncontrollably while trying to focus on tasks that involved folding paper and working with blocks. She could only assume that she had failed the test, because she was next taken to a ward in the girls' home. There she discovered kids who, like her, were mostly just normal teens from impoverished and troubled backgrounds. Yet they too were considered to be mentally defective.

The children with whom she shared this fate were not just

imprisoned, they were bullied, dehumanized, physically brutalized, and sexually assaulted by attendants and older inmates. Some were used as subjects in experiments. Doris's brother Albert would later recall being selected to be in a "science club," whose young members were, unbeknownst to them, fed hot cereal laced with radioactive calcium. This was part of an experiment sponsored by Harvard University, MIT, the Atomic Energy Commission, and Quaker Oats. Other forms of nonconsensual medicalized interventions at these institutions included lobotomy, electroshock therapy, and surgical sterilization.

Like other higher-functioning children at the institution, Doris was eventually enrolled in the labor force of inmates who were put in charge of running the facility as a cost-saving measure. She had to clean and take care of younger and less abled children. The responsibility she found the most grueling was caring for the most disabled kids on the premises. She recalled having to spoon-feed them through the bars of cages. She was too scared to open the door because they would try to grab her. Some appeared so misshapen that she forgot they were human, and she was worried that whatever justified their confinement might be contagious. She was not sure why they had been singled out to be caged. She was paralyzed with fear, worried she would be next.

After living the horrors of Fernald for four years, Doris felt compelled to choose between family and survival, loyalty and escape. She decided to run to survive. During her next visit with her brothers, she told them she was planning her escape. She promised she would one day come back for them, but for now, she was running away.

The date would become etched in her memory. It was the first Sunday in July 1952 when she went back to her room and changed for her long journey the way only a teenager would, by putting on shorts and a T-shirt. When the coast was clear, she slipped out. Doris had been working as a maid in the superintendent's house and was under less strict supervision. She walked to the main road and stuck out her thumb. She jumped in the first car that stopped. The young driver's destination was Buffalo, a town about which she knew nothing. She did not hesitate. Anyplace was going to be better than Fernald.

When they arrived in the border city, the young man, a soldier who had made a pass at her but thankfully had taken no for an answer, explained that he would be going on to Canada and could not take her along. She had no papers, and he was not willing to risk getting in trouble with the authorities. He dropped her off at the Peace Bridge, which connects Buffalo to Fort Erie, Ontario. Doris was alone and penniless in a place where she knew nothing and no one, but she finally felt free.

After the gruesome tale that had preceded it, the account of Doris's escape to Buffalo was such a relief that I somehow expected a happily-ever-after ending, even in attenuated form. Surely she had experienced enough heartache, I thought. Surely fate, life, or chance would finally give her a break. But Doris seemed destined to bear more than her fair share of misfortune in a lifetime. Sometimes, when trauma goes on begetting more trauma, life feels less believable than fiction.

On the fateful July day when she was dropped off in downtown Buffalo, Doris was so destitute that she wandered into the first church she saw. It was a Catholic church, whose priest would arrange to find her a place at a home for girls called the House of the Good Shepherd. There, the nuns listened to her story and, not finding it believable, arranged for her to be examined at a local psychiatric hospital. Doris felt like she had no choice but to comply. She was deemed sane. The health-care professionals there contacted the authorities in Massachusetts to see whether she should be returned. The answer came back in the affirmative, but Doris was fortunately then of a legal age in New York State to be able to make her own decisions. She chose to stay in Buffalo. Arrangements were made for her to become a live-in caretaker for an elderly blind woman, whose son Doris would eventually marry when she turned eighteen. He was thirty-five years old.

Doris remembered being traumatized by her wedding night: "I didn't know anything [about sex]. I never had a young life." She later discovered that her betrothed was sterile, which would eventually provide the grounds for the annulment of the marriage. She subsequently met her second husband, James, an autoworker with whom she had six children.

Tragically, Doris's second marriage was no more fulfilling than her first. James refused to give her any money, not even to run the household, so she decided to become a state-certified caregiver for mentally disabled individuals, to whom she could attend in her own home. Not only did she need the income to put food on the table, but her husband had forbidden her to work outside the home. The love in the name of which she had gotten remarried was once again exposed as a lie.

For twenty years, she endured her husband's emotional abuse, until she reached a point of no return. She took him out to a lobster dinner and told him in the safety of a restaurant's public setting that she was leaving him. Her youngest child was twelve years old, the age at which Doris had been separated from her foster family and institutionalized. She did not look back to consider that she was restaging the abandonment she had suffered as a child. That would have assumed a sense of power and authority she had never had. She was yet again in survival mode.

Several years later, Doris's subsequent relationship was so physically abusive that a family court judge who was handling her case called her to the bench to recommend she buy a gun and learn to use it if she wanted to stay alive. Justice would only be served when a virulent cancer finally took Doris's third husband mere weeks after his diagnosis.

Doris's past was marked by such relentless tragedies that her inability to love, which had first struck me as bordering on the absurd, now felt inevitable. Trust, the foundation on which love and the ability to feel it are built, had been shattered by a lifetime of betrayals. The serial abuse, abandonment, and confinement she had experienced had all been inflicted by people who had professed to love her and the caretakers who ultimately failed her. Even her closest familial bonds, first with her mother and brothers, and then with her own children, had left her with gaping holes. Doris confessed that her inability to develop emotional attachment had even defined her relationship with her children. As a young mother, she had always felt as if she was performing a duty; she had certainly fed her kids, taken care of them, and treated them well, but she had done so like an automaton. She knew to say "I love you" but did not feel it. She was all business. Her relationship with her little ones was missing a fundamental ingredient.

I no longer wondered why she was who she was or why her end-of-life experiences were so impersonal. In her own words, Doris "could not give back" what she "had not received."

Maybe it was not just that love had failed her; maybe she felt as if she had failed love. Despite her promise to her brothers, Doris had never been able to go back for them. She had been too scared to reenter Massachusetts. By the time she reunited with her siblings, much later in life, it was too late. They were more strangers to one another than family. Similarly, giving up custody of her kids when she left her second husband had led to her estrangement from them later. By the time I met Doris, they were back in touch, but their communication felt stilted to her.

I asked Doris about her dreams again. I was hoping that maybe she'd had new ones and that reviewing them might help her reconnect with what she could hold dear.

Pre-death dreams and visions are much more discriminating than the saying "We die as we live" may intimate. They do not appropriate past events wholesale. While summoning up familiar territory, they cut out distressing elements, embellish empowering ones, and provide the dying person with the visions and re-visions they most need to make a peaceful transition. They may stage the reliving of a trauma, but it is typically in such a way as to transcend its debilitating effects.

This is when Doris shared her more recent dream, one that answered the question that had been preoccupying me: How can one walk through life devoid of the feeling of love? It turns out that one can't, and one doesn't.

Unbeknownst to her, Doris's first dream, the one about flying, had addressed her two most pressing but also paradoxical needs: the need to be freed from all she knew and the need to be loved. Life may not have provided her with any outlets for the satisfaction of these two contradictory impulses, but her end-of-life experiences did, even summoning an angel as a symbol of the love she had previously forsaken.

Doris did not want to die before "I know for sure that I am saved by grace. I want to know that I am saved before I go." I asked her how she would know. "Because the Bible says so," she replied with aplomb. A born-again Christian, Doris believed that her first dream was "preparing me in a way. It is kind of like a warning to me, to make sure I am ready" because "I have been dreaming since I have been sick." Then, with the impish expression with which she qualified all her graver statements, she added, "The devil does not want me, so the Lord has to take me. He is stuck with me, you see, and I know he loves me; I know he loves me." Doris uttered these words in pure excitement, waving her arms as if she were dancing to the rhythmic cadence of her own words. In her exuberance, she was finally able to identify a source of love in her life. It was a form of abstract love, but it was love all the same—one she finally thought she deserved.

I asked Doris how she interpreted that first dream. My question was immediately met with a rebuff: "I don't know what it means. Who are the other people? Strangers, no one that I know, people I don't know. I told them don't be afraid, I am here flying over there." Then she entertained a possible interpretation: "I moved a lot, so maybe I am moving again. I never stayed in one place long. Like, I want to move from here. Why do I feel like I have to be moving all the time? Why can I not feel at home? Settle down? Like it is home, you know." I asked her when she had first started dreaming about flying ("Not too long ago") and how old she was in her dream. "I was younger than this. I can't really say but I know I was not this old. I was always running; I wanted to be free. But free from what? I had six children!"

Doris seemed as confused as I was by the underlying meaning of what she was experiencing. She dismissed the idea that her dream could have been about freedom at a time in her life when she could not have divested herself of her maternal responsibilities. Still, although the meaning was not really intelligible to her, the impact was palpable. In fact, what mattered to her was not what the dream meant but the feeling it evoked. When I finally inquired if the vision had felt real, she answered, "At the time it did. I would have liked it to be. I was laying here, and I thought it was real." She may not have known exactly what it meant, but she knew how it felt. She was more comfortable detached and freed from the cruel promise of human connection. Unbound by the demands of worldly love, she was dying as she had lived, by escaping, only now it was by taking refuge in her religious beliefs.

Her second recurring dream was even more poignant. She dreamed of Richard, her last long-term relationship, the only man who had neither physically nor verbally abused her.

They had gotten together on a whim. He was a "looker" and always made sure that he was dressed to the nines. They both vowed that their relationship was based on mere physical attraction. Their deliberate lack of commitment kept their involvement light and airy, and before she knew it, they had been together for fourteen years, in playfulness and unaccountability but also in sickness and in health. Then one day, Richard suggested they radically change the terms of their relationship. He asked for her hand in marriage. Doris not only refused; she did what she had always done: escaped. This time, however, she did so by telling her partner of more than a decade that they would soon be moving to a new home, which he took to be a prelude to married life. She set him up in "their" new apartment in the small town of Batavia, New York, an hour away from her home, and disappeared without leaving a forwarding address. He tried contacting her for a while, to no avail.

Now, more than twenty years after she left him, and five years after she heard of his passing, Doris was dreaming of Richard. The man she had previously described as overly fashion-minded, with hair primped and eyebrows tweezed, was now looking at her in her dream as he had never done before. He was gentle, and he held her gaze with a beseeching expression that moved her. He approached her with outstretched arms, ready to receive her in the most heartfelt embrace. He appeared "like he really wanted me, that he wanted me purely," she explained in a tone that spelled both disbelief and revelation. She could hear his voice whisper, "I love you."

The person she had once rejected in distrust was now claiming her love. Her end-of-life experiences dramatized and amplified the glimmer of love she had once received from this man whose living counterpart had displayed such self-absorption. But in her dreams, he was apologizing; they were talking, laughing, dancing, and reconnecting in ways that were unlike him in the flesh. She woke up feeling much warmth, with her heart beating excitedly, and hoping she could go back to sleep to resume her rekindled romance.

Thanks to her end-of-life experiences, Doris was getting a second chance, a final opportunity to expose herself to the vulnerability that love ultimately demands. There may have been little love in the databank of Doris's reality, but her end-of-life dreams were finally giving her what her lived experiences and relationships had denied her. And in that moment, what mattered more than any exact correspondence between Richard's feelings in life and the ones she imagined now was her new-found ability to feel love. The important point was not whether the love she was conjuring in her dreams was true to what had actually transpired. What mattered was that she was finally capable of heeding its call and exhibiting a receptiveness to human attachment she had not dared risk before. Her pre-death dreams and visions fulfilled the emotional needs that her life had consistently failed to meet. She was freed from pathological attachments, constraints, and abuse in one dream and could finally experience love in the other.

Doris may never have gotten over the extreme difficulty she had in trusting or building relationships in life, but after these dreams, she ventured that "Richard may have been the first person who truly loved me. For me." She was at last able to reclaim and see herself as worthy of the love her younger self had pushed away. I knew enough about Doris to realize that this was the closest she would ever get to a declaration of love. After all, love received is the inevitable precursor to love given.

More dramatically than anyone I knew, Doris managed at life's end to draw on the broken fragments of her unbearable past in order to reassemble herself into wholeness. She re-created the love that her life experiences had not given her but that, despite her overly insistent denial, she'd had the capacity to feel all along. She soothed her deep wounds and did more healing and growth in the last months of her life than she had ever been able to do in the course of her long existence. Her journey, as does Dwayne's, suggests that the mark of our humanity may reside in this extraordinary potential for transformation at life's end, a final rally to fight injustice, heal old wounds, and restore a love that was once damaged or withheld.

For me, Doris was also the patient whose dreams most explicitly demonstrated the importance of looking at end-of-life experiences as a process that takes place in the context of someone's past and present relationships, and not in isolation from them. Pre-death dreams and visions are not singular entities with singular and fixed meanings. They do not constitute an ingredient that can be added near death to produce a predetermined outcome. In fact, they would be meaningless outside the relationships and trajectories that define each patient's life. Their meanings and effects are unique to the life lived. What is experienced as liberating by one person may be excruciating to another. That was true, for instance, for my friend Patty, whose pre-death dreams of flying and moving were as distressing to her as they were freeing to Doris.

It was not just her fellow officers at the Buffalo Police Department who were grief-stricken when Officer Patty Parete was shot in the line of duty. It was the entire Buffalo community. The incident occurred on the night of December 5, 2006, when Patty and her partner, Carl Andolina, responded to a fight call at a convenience store. When they approached the scene, they were shot by an eighteen-year-old boy who feared being sent to prison now that he was of legal age and was no longer eligible for youthful offender status. Patty was shot twice, point-blank. The first bullet struck her bulletproof vest, but the second one went through her chin, traveling through her body to lodge itself in her spine. Patty was left paralyzed from the neck down. She was forty-one.

After the shooting, members of the Buffalo Police Department kept a vigil at her hospital bedside, while the Upstate New York community rallied to raise over half a million dollars for her care. Patty underwent rehabilitation at the Kessler Institute for Rehabilitation in West Orange, New Jersey, but after nine months of physical therapy, she was still unable to move her arms and legs. In 2009, a new custom-designed, handicap-accessible house was built for her in Niagara County, and the city of Buffalo worked out an unprecedented deal to pay salary and benefits to her life partner and caregiver, Mary Ellen.

For Mary Ellen, becoming Patty's full-time caretaker meant quitting the job she loved as a pediatric ICU nurse. Other friends rallied to provide the couple with the help and resources they needed. After Patty's release from the hospital, complete strangers, including celebrities, would often ask to meet with her to express their appreciation and support. It was not that Patty was not grateful for these outpourings of emotional and material support. She was. On good days, she would even express it. The problem was that her good days were so few and far between that, unlike Doris, she wanted to die. Or rather, as she told me again and again, she didn't want to live but was too afraid to die.

What Patty feared most was less death itself than what would happen were she to decide not to go on living. Even though her faith had been shaken to the core by the horror she was experiencing, Patty obsessed about the afterlife. Would she be doomed to eternal damnation? Would her soul be trapped in purgatory? How could God, if there was one, not know that her endurance had reached its limits? Would she who had run out of hope truly never be forgiven?

It was because of the severity of her physical symptoms that I was asked to take her on as a patient. Her bodily pain, which was rivaled only by the depth of her psychological suffering, was excruciating. She had no feeling below the neck, yet she experienced phantom sensations, medically defined as a central pain syndrome, and it felt, as she put it, "like being dipped in burning oil."

On her best days, Patty was notoriously hard on doctors, so at first, my involvement in her care felt like being picked out of a lineup. I mean this in the most respectful and loving way: Patty was an extraordinarily difficult and stubborn patient. She would not be patronized by anybody, not even the medical professional on whose expertise her comfort and life depended. Early in our relationship, Patty began referring to me as "my doctor." I was touched. The phrase sounded personalizing, almost endearing. But it wasn't long before she began telling me what to do, what not to do, and how to do it. I soon realized that the expression "my doctor" was more of a possessive statement than tender gesture. She owned me and made it clear. In a sense, she gave me permission to be her doctor. And as if to prove it, she once fired me, then hired me back, as if on a whim, bluntly claiming that I was "a keeper."

Patty had been repeatedly hurt by what she had experienced as an abandonment of sorts, when her doctors came and went. After a particularly frustrating exchange, one of the many that erupted from her deep-rooted suspicion and distrust, I finally scribbled a few lines on a piece of paper and held our new "contract" in front of her. It read, "I, *Your* Doctor, will not abandon you, Patty Parete. Ever." Patty kept that handwritten note in the drawer of her night table and insisted it travel with her whenever she had to go to the hospital. Those were now the written yet unspoken terms of our relationship, and neither of us ever felt the need to revisit them.

Patty suffered. She suffered like no patient I had ever had, and like no one ever should. I did what I could to lessen the suffering, and she did what she could to end it. She constantly begged me, her nurses, and her lifelong partner to help her die.

The degree of pain she had to endure, both physically and psychologically, was so extreme that it led to as high a turnover among the hired help as among her doctors. The secondary trauma experienced by caretakers in the presence of someone in severe and unremitting distress cannot be underestimated. Tragically, Patty's refusal to engage with life beyond her room eventually pushed her partner, Mary Ellen, away. Polly, a dear friend of many years, moved in to oversee the difficult task of managing Patty's care.

Patty struggled more and more with her growing dependency on the mechanical ventilator that regulated her breathing at night. The bedtime ritual of being placed on the machine caused the most discomfort, physically and psychologically, and the battles between patient and caregivers worsened. Patty's oxygen levels would drop, alarms would go off to indicate the urgent need for the ventilator to sustain life, while Patty begged, yelled, and demanded to be left at peace.

For years, her dreams provided no relief. If anything, they were a source of misery, and she woke from them more upset and tormented than before. Dreaming often meant seeing herself as the able-bodied and active person she would never be again. She would dream of skydiving, of soaring through the air while defying gravity. She could feel the rush of cold wind that filled the airplane right before she jumped, the goosebumps that rose across her arms and neck at watching the landscape unfold beneath her. More often, she dreamt of riding her beloved motorcycle. She felt its power between her legs as she sped down wide-open country roads. She could smell the trees, grass, hay, and the exhaust. She relived the adrenaline-fueled, hyperaware emotional state that came with the ride. But these dreams also meant that she was forced to wake up and confront the discordant reality of her injury and its gruesome limits. Her distress was intense and unrelenting as she kept revisiting the collision between what she experienced with her eyes open and closed.

Patty never adapted to her circumstances. She saw her limitations as a violation of her right to choose, live, be, and even breathe freely. Acceptance was simply not an option. She adamantly refused to entertain, let alone accept, the idea of her body as disabled. It wasn't that she didn't have the mental fortitude to do so, she just neither had the will nor the intention. Her injury and its forced compromise were an affront to her and antithetical to everything she stood for. Her life had been marked by sheer physicality, competence, and independence, and she was not about to reimagine it any other way.

This was a woman with a passion for the outdoors, for running, and for her Harley-Davidson V-Rod motorcycle. Her bike had truly been an expression of who she was. She had customized it—with ghost flames against a purple backdrop—to make it uniquely hers, and although she enjoyed the Harley mystique, she had not fallen for it hook, line, and sinker. In fact, she had made a point of trading her Harley 883 Sportster for the anniversary year V-Rod model, which, to many aficionados, did not really feel or sound like a Harley. But Patty did not care. She did not feel the need to prove her credentials, not even to the Harley community she loved. She would ride with a handpicked group of women ("Don't ask, can't join") up and down the streets of Buffalo, and she would rev the throttle so loudly that the sound would set off car alarms on the vehicles parked along the way.

Patty was not one to surrender her core strength. Her firmness could be rigid at times, but it also functioned as a form of moral principle—her principle, one that drove her to be utterly fair and completely unbending. She would never have let circumstances diminish her fearless determination, had it not been for the debilitating spinal injury that destroyed her life.

Patty had joined the police force in 2001, at age thirty-six. For the next five years, she had maintained peak physical fitness through unparalleled commitment and focus. Few if any of her colleagues could boast of having "nearly zero percent body fat" as she did. Like Eddie, who had retired from the same police force because of his compromised physical condition, she was conscious of the ways in which her fitness, or lack thereof, could affect her ability to fulfill her duty as an officer. She considered physical prowess paramount to her ability to do her job and do it well.

In the midst of the tragedy she experienced as an irreversible rupture, Patty nonetheless remained the same person she had always been. She was still as difficult as she was charming, as tender as she was tough, as frugal in words as she was rich in meaning. She was often distant, even aloof, yet at the same time completely aware. She followed the details of the lives that surrounded her, sharing in her friends' daily concerns and joys and celebrating their accomplishments. She always had an opinion about everyone and everything, from people's relationships to their dressing habits. And she did not mince her words. With one pointed look, she could size you up, and she could call you out. I remember her wicked sense of humor. I still see her pirate smile. I will never forget the time I suggested she name her new Chihuahua after me—Chris, or CJ for Chris Jr. Patty just smiled, slowly, and told me she would consider it. A few weeks later, I asked about the dog. She gave me one of her pirate smiles and said, "Do you mean Jerry? He was just at the vet, getting fixed." I was confounded, and she was amused.

Animals touched her in a very special way. Patty left her house only three times in the last two years of her life, twice to come to my horse farm. On these occasions, we would leave her alone in a stall with a horse named Chancellor. He never left her side and stood with his head above hers, hardly moving. We would place hay on her lap, and Chancellor would gently grab a few strands at a time.

As many horses do, Chancellor liked to dip his hay in water before chewing. So, we would deliberately place his water bucket beside Patty's wheelchair. She would close her eyes, tilt her head back, and feel the water drops on her face as the magnificent and gentle horse stood and ate alongside her. She remained silent.

Patty never looked more at peace than on these days she spent in my barn. She had made a connection that made sense to her. It made sense to me too. Chancellor was no ordinary horse. At seventeen hands, he was huge, he was beautiful, and he was the grandson of the greatest horse of them all, Secretariat. Like all great horses, Secretariat, "the horse that God built," knew how special he was. He was physically striking and brave, and he ran faster than any horse that had ever lived. He ran because that's who he was; it felt right, and it was just in him. Patty was like that too. Courageous, uncompromising, beautiful, and most alive when she was at her most physical.

Over time, Patty's health deteriorated. She was more and more dependent on the mechanical ventilator even during the day. As she drew closer to the reality of death, her fears—about abandonment, suffering, and the afterlife—faded. She stopped dreaming of her life before her injury or mulling over her irrecoverable loss. She no longer awoke to unimaginable terror. Instead, her thoughts went to a renewed concern for others. She talked openly about those who had sacrificed so much for her care over the years, Mary Ellen and Polly, whose gift of love she could never repay. Her fear of death lessened, and in its place emerged expressions of love that had been buried within the depths of her suffering.

In her pre-death dreams, Patty was now finally embraced by the one who had loved her first, and would love her last—her mom, Dorothea. She had never stopped mourning the loss of her mother, often expressing her longing to be reunited with the parent she had lost three years earlier. Whereas dreaming of restored bodily movements had previously been a source of pain upon waking, the soul-lifting sensation of being hugged and hugging back now stayed with her and carried over into her other relationships. She was now able to recognize the deep loyalty and commitment her friends had shown her. She saw their sacrifice not as a symptom of the burden she felt she was but as a sign of their grace and humanity; she could voice the deep gratitude she felt. I was reminded of chaplain Kerry Egan's beautiful words: "The first, and usually the last, classroom of love is the family." Patty's end-of-life experiences put her back in touch with the familiar and familial love she needed to be able to transcend her tragic circumstances and to finally reach a gentle acceptance and love.

Illness may have turned her inward, but at death's door, Patty, who had struggled with expressions of tenderness her entire life, was now seeing the pain of others—mine included. Before she died, she motioned for me to get close, like she always did, with subtle movements of her face. As I drew near to lend her my ear, she kissed me, her doctor, "my doctor," and said, "I love you." She was not saying good-bye so much as tending to me, the greatest gesture of empathy I have experienced as a doctor.

Patty passed that evening.

Since the horrible day of the shooting, Patty had been surrounded by love and unparalleled acts of friendship. I was privileged to witness the remarkable kindness, devotion, and grace she summoned in the loved ones who worked selflessly to ease her suffering. Every day, her hair was lovingly brushed, her cheeks were kissed, and her unfeeling hand was held. She was never abandoned, never alone. It was in those moments and in those simple gestures that goodness and love triumphed over tragedy. What arose from an inconceivable loss were lessons of giving, empathy, and uncommon love that transcended the limitations of her injury and illness. We learned that people continue to have worth even when they are not the same as they once were. Patty was cherished to the end. This was the meaning of the unconditional love her friends had embodied and that she could finally recognize. Seeing herself reunited with her long-lost mother was her solace and the final enactment of the justice others had sought in retribution.

When Helen Keller was told that death is no more than passing from one room into another, she signed, "But there is a difference for me, you know, because in that room, I should be able to see." My hope is that Patty found "that room" too, one in which she could feel whole again.

At life's end, people's stories often come to the surface in surprising ways. I witnessed as both Doris and Patty freed themselves from confinement before reaching love and wholeness. Doris broke free to fly above a hurtful world and in the end, she felt the presence of the love she had been denied. Patty transcended her injuries by reaching back to a familiar maternal love. She could finally feel concern for more than her own tragic circumstances and be grateful for her friends' anchoring presence. Both women were released from the severe limitations that had constrained their existence, but not without an unfathomable struggle.

If there is accomplishment in dying it is a transcendent one, but not in a way that would be reserved for the spiritual and religious. A spiritual death is what I believe both Doris and Patty had, one that summoned hard work and courage. That may truly be our only path to wholeness and happiness at life's end. It is a process of the heart, and through end-of-life experiences, it takes us beyond our known limits, creating openness where there sometimes was none. It signifies less the end of life than its affirmation and embrace.

# love
# knows
# no
# limits

*Love knows no limits, but ardently transcends all bounds.*
*Love feels no burden, takes no account of toil, attempts things*
*beyond its strength.*

—THOMAS À KEMPIS

As an ordained priest writing a devotional text in the fifteenth century, Thomas à Kempis wanted to define the uniqueness of Christ's love for humanity. Similarly, for the influential thirteenth-century Persian poet Rūmī, "to love is to reach God." What I have found at the bedside of dying patients is that the boundlessness these theologians ascribe to divine love also defines how my patients express and experience love in their end-of-life dreams. Sometimes, patients' love for their deceased "better half" is such a defining feature of their identity that it remains a vital lived experience after their partner passes. It also becomes a constant feature of their end-of-life dreams and visions. This is often true for those who face death together after decades of a shared life. It is the kind of limitless love that outlasts the death of a beloved in such an uncompromising way that its story trickles down the generations, through family lore and stories, myths and poems, and books such as this one.

Yet when we think about romantic love, the love shared by elderly couples is one we hardly hear about. Old love, like old age, is not romantic, or so we are led to believe. That is because relationships that are typically hailed as the pinnacle of romance have everything to do with youth, vibrancy, and brevity. Think of Shakespeare's star-crossed lovers Romeo and Juliet, the universal icons of romantic love. As my patient Patricia—a self-proclaimed Shakespeare aficionado (her word)—once remarked, Romeo and Juliet met at sixteen and thirteen, respectively, and knew each other for the whole of four days before deciding to spend the rest of their lives together or die trying. The lives of older couples, let alone dying couples, are rarely the kind of stories that are evoked when we think of romantic love.

Yet the epitome of love may be seen when older couples who have been married for fifty-plus years come in, holding hands and exchanging loving glances. Dying has a way of bringing into focus the strength of people's love, and few love stories are more romantic than that of two old souls who no longer finish each other's sentences, because they don't have to. I recognize it when I ask for their stories, and although they have yet to inspire a bestseller, what I get in return is an account of true love, one that outlasts life, permeates their end-of-life dreams, and seeps into their waking reality. It is in the end-of-life experiences of the dying that one can often recognize the purest expression of love.

⁂

"My memory starts and ends with him." These words were spoken by the wife of a hospice patient, whom I met about fifteen years ago. Alizah was seventy-four years old and tending to her dying husband, her partner of fifty-four years. I had seen the many faces of grief in hospice, but her appearance of consuming pain and shock stopped me in my tracks. "I have not known of a life without him," she whispered. I still remember where she was standing when she uttered those words. I remember her meek demeanor and beseeching eyes, her look of utter despair.

I listened speechless when Alizah told me about meeting Nathan, a love story that belonged as much in history books as in a personal narrative.

Their story began on October 21, 1942, in Szczebrzeszyn, Poland, on the fateful day during World War II when the occupying Germans rounded up the Jews in the village. Alizah was thirteen years old. Along with neighbors and other townsfolk, her family had been driven from their home and ordered to assemble in the marketplace. There were hundreds of men, women, and children, stunned and fear-stricken, all lined up in rows. In the midst of the shouting and frequent gunfire, Alizah could hardly register the surreal events that were unraveling before her eyes. Her childhood friend Nathan, a fifteen-year-old neighborhood boy, stood in an alleyway, watching in horror as those he loved were being taken.

Out of the corner of her eye, Alizah saw Nathan run toward her. He grabbed her hand and pulled her from the lineup. She instinctively knew that he was dragging her to safety, and miraculously, they escaped notice in the chaos of the day. It was, she described, as if the two of them were moving in a parallel universe where time had stopped.

Alizah would never see her relatives again, and it would be some time before she learned of their gruesome end at the Belzec death camp, a fate from which Nathan had saved her.

The two teens survived the war in hiding and went on to be adopted by American families, reuniting years later. They would eventually get married and live full lives. Together, these remaining fragments of two decimated families reconstituted the sense of wholeness that had been shattered by the genocidal war.

Now, as Alizah sat by Nathan's bedside, holding his hand, she could not fathom facing the world without him. To her, he was everybody and everything all rolled in one, the tie that bound her to a past that nobody but he could possibly understand. He was her life.

All I could offer them was my presence and a desire to bear witness, while knowing full well that even offering empathy would feel shallow. Nathan's inner life contained depths of tragedy and strength that were beyond my comprehension and reach, a harsh reminder that some wounds, particularly old ones, can never be healed or soothed. Alizah was the embodiment of their shared history and inseparability, and Nathan's dying experience was lived outwardly through her.

As a doctor, I was of limited help to Nathan, but I felt compelled to comfort Alizah. Watching her interact with him reminded me that people who have received and given love never die alone. At no time did the importance of treating the person in the bed by caring for those they love resonate more fully. I could not reach him, but I knew she could. After all, as a boy, he had risked his life to rescue a thirteen-year-old girl from certain death, and I knew that this same soul, now within an old and dying body, would take solace in knowing that Alizah was comforted.

Having witnessed death as atrocity, Alizah would have been unable to envision dying as a peaceful process had Nathan not shown her how. He was once again the person who guided her through the inconceivable. He taught her about dreaming while dying, just like he had once taught her about surviving while grieving. As Nathan's life neared its end, his dreams reverted not to the trauma of their youth but to the soothing memories of his lost family. His distant past returned to him after a lifetime of fighting to repress all recollection of it. Surviving the Holocaust had meant forgoing looking back or fully grieving. As his family's sole survivor, he had felt his life was both a gift and a burden, a reminder of the inescapable responsibility to live for those whose lives had been taken. If he managed to move on, it was by placing one foot in front of the other, one step at a time, with Alizah by his side. Now, as he lay dying, his burden was lifted and his mind could safely drift to the gentle recesses of his past, a time of true childhood innocence, before the atrocities. His dead relatives returned to him, safe and together again. And he was able to share his end-of-life experiences with Alizah, the only person who could truly understand the weight of such a past. It took dying for Nathan to reacquaint himself with his family and all that was once familiar. And it took seeing the peace and serenity with which Nathan approached life's end for Alizah to rally spiritually.

According to ancient Chinese lore, there is a "red string of fate" that connects people who are destined to meet, regardless of time, place, or circumstance. It may stretch or tangle, but it will never break. Alizah's life and well-being was so interwoven with Nathan's, their connection so palpable and strong, I would not have been surprised to discover around their ankles the silken thread with which the god of love in Chinese mythology is said to bind predestined couples.

One of the greatest privileges of my role as a doctor has been to witness the life stage that summons the very best in people, the qualities that they are often unaware they possess: courage, strength, grace, and selflessness in the face of loss. It is like a stress test that, rather than measuring the heart's biological function, reveals the immeasurable depth of its capacity for love. And it is a test that requires no electrodes to detect and convey the rhythms and scope of lifelong romance. Dying has a way of defining and amalgamating the depth of those feelings with an intensity few stories illustrate better than those of my patients. This is true of Alizah and Nathan's remarkable story, as well as of widowed patients whose lifelong relationship, although cut short by the death of their loved one, remains their most sustaining source of support during the dying process. These are stories that reveal extraordinary people and moments in the most ordinary lives. My patients may not be young or restless, but to me, the love stories of Patricia and Chuck, Benny and Gloria, Joan and Sonny, and Beverly and Bill, whom you'll meet next, resonate just as powerfully as any young and intense romance. These couples are no less moving or romantic than history's most iconic lovers.

For the elderly couples I have cared for at Hospice Buffalo, being separated by death after a lifetime of togetherness is simply not an option. After losing their other half, the surviving partner will do what they have to do to stay whole: keep their loved one alive, consciously or unconsciously, through stories and memories, and maybe most vividly through their pre-death dreams, daily and relentlessly.

When Patricia remembered or dreamed about her deceased husband, Chuck, it was not as a ninety-year-old dying patient with a terminal disease and compromised mobility. It was with the rapture of a younger mind and healthy body, weightless and carefree, still able to walk, and full of anticipation for what the future holds: "I'd like to wake up and walk up to Chuck and take him by the hand and walk into the eternal sunset."

They met when Patricia was just fifteen and he nineteen, two months before he went off to war. "I knew I was going to marry him—I know this sounds like a fairy tale—within weeks of meeting him," she explained. "I loved him more than life itself. We knew, we knew then that we would end up together and never ever considered anyone else. I love him to this day more than I love anything. He was wonderful, funny, smart, and curious, perfect . . . and so kind, sweet."

As Patricia was nearing the end of her life, the man of her dreams fittingly became the man in her dreams. Like most end-of-life experiences, Patricia's encapsulated the essence of their relationship even though very little was said. They were a simple but beautiful tribute to their lives together. "I used to go to the Cazenovia pool every day to swim," she recounted, "and my husband would take a walk at South Park botanical gardens. He'd get home first, and every day when I'd get home, he'd have the tea ready, and the crossword puzzle. He always wore white T-shirts with the sleeves. Gleaming white T-shirts. He was standing there, and I remember saying, 'God, you're still a good-looking guy.' I remember thinking that, and he just smiled and said, 'Hi.' Then it dissolves. I was with him for a minute or two, and it was nice. These are very happy dreams. They feel wonderful for me. They're going back to something real. It's love. A tiny little thing, but love."

It was in the context of this "tiny little thing" called love that Patricia felt the most sustained. So it was not surprising that it was to the ordinary, day-to-day experience of living with Chuck, such as solving crossword puzzles, that her pre-death dreams returned, again and again.

> Charles would read the puzzles, and I would give the
> answer, and he would write. I never thought about that. He
> could provide some answers—I let him—I didn't take over
> that much. He was a smart man, and he could have done a
> lot of them, but it was easier for him to write than to think
> about it. What a faker you were, Charles.

I was particularly touched when Patricia paused to address her late husband by name. She was neither confused nor dreaming at that point. The statement was uttered as if she were talking to herself. We have all caught ourselves uttering things out loud that we believe we were just thinking to ourselves. Patricia's aside was just such a moving testimony to the intimacy she still shared with her husband years after his death. The love she felt had no temporal boundaries. She described an afternoon as "being with him for a minute or two." Dying is about living in a timeless dreamworld where visions of the departed are more real than the reality that exists outwardly without them. It is a world where love does not need to be incarnated to be felt, or unexamined to be unconditional.

Grieving patients who face death do not fear or adulate it; they just wait for it.

It is true that everyone will have come across the story of an old couple who died within days of each other. I have known many. I met people who followed their partner into death in the absence of any clear medical prognosis. We all knew that it was due to a broken heart, and that this was neither a metaphor nor a romanticized assessment. It is now established as medical fact that a real-life broken heart can lead to cardiac consequences. The medical diagnosis has a name: broken-heart syndrome, or in medical parlance, stress-induced or takotsubo cardiomyopathy. It usually happens quietly, surreptitiously, with no further ado.

A broken heart best describes what happened to ninety-year-old Bernard—Benny to his loved ones—shortly after his wife Gloria's passing. At the time of Gloria's death, Benny had been in good health. At eighty-seven, he was active, gregarious, and independent, visiting a lifetime's worth of friends and family. He loved to drive, and did so daily around Buffalo, the town in which he had lived his whole life. After Gloria's precipitous death from an infection, he was inconsolable. He kept wishing for an early death, imploring God to let him rejoin his "Glo."

Benny would visit the cemetery daily, sometimes up to three times a day. There, he would sit or kneel in front of Gloria's gravestone, praying and talking to her, resurrecting her in memory. When his daughter Maureen tried to dissuade him from prostrating himself, his rebuke was immediate. "To each his own," he answered.

On Valentine's Day 2016, exactly two months after Gloria's passing, Benny insisted on sticking to his daily routine despite subzero temperatures. When Maureen arrived at the cemetery, she could not refrain from asking the question whose answer she knew too well: "What are you trying to do? Kill yourself?" Benny did not miss a beat: "I could only wish." This is the same man who had found it in himself to tell his dying wife that it was "okay to let go now." But it wasn't, not then, not now, not ever.

On that fateful day, with temperatures plummeting to minus 15, Maureen found her father walking around Gloria's tombstone. He looked like he was going around in circles, resolute and heavy-footed as he worked his way through the snow. From a distance, she first assumed it was the cold that kept him moving, but she soon noticed that he was walking in too deliberate a pattern and was retracing his steps. As she drew closer, she saw that he had been carving a heart in the snow around her grave.

Benny was usually solemn and reflective after his visits to the cemetery. Things were different that evening. He appeared breathless and uncomfortable. His status worsened over the next forty-eight hours, and by the time he was taken to the emergency room, he was critically ill. He was diagnosed with having suffered a heart attack that had been stuttering over the past few days. Benny's heart literally broke on Valentine's Day.

The absence of immediate medical intervention had caused an irreversible heart condition that required hospice care. In the space of forty-eight hours, Benny had gone from being fully independent to being unable to fend for himself. He had to move in with his daughter. He could no longer visit Gloria's grave, so he began to visit her in his dreams. Or, as his daughter evocatively stated, "He is living in his dreams now." She could hear him at night, singing to his beloved Gloria in Polish, the shared language of their upbringing. This once overly social man would awake only briefly to eat, preferring to return to bed so he could close his eyes and revisit his wife.

Old couples have much to teach us about true love. Their bond requires no big declarations, loyalty tests, or dramatic endings. It just needs and takes time. It unravels and infuses every fiber of their being, so much so that they cannot conceive of living without it. And so they don't. They move on through life's obstacles with the certainty of its existence. They continue to feel and believe in it even when the person through whom that love originated leaves them. For elderly patients especially, their love for their other half is who they are. Job, ambition, hobbies, mortgage, and plans have come and gone. What is left and what matters is the relationships they have maintained, cherished, and tended to through a lifetime of small gestures and greetings, loving glances and humorous words, shared stories and forgiven faults.

It may be that our cultural representations of romantic love have it all wrong. Love at its best, deepest, and strongest is not about youth, impulsivity, drama, or despair. It is about constancy, patience, trust, forgiveness, and sustained acceptance. It is about letting go of the living and not letting go of the dead.

After fifty-seven years of marriage, Joan and Alfred's love colored all the dreams and visions Joan had during the two months that preceded their reunion in death. Joan and the man she had affectionately nicknamed Sonny were also born to first-generation Polish immigrants. Their families settled across the street from one another in a working-class suburb of Buffalo, where they grew up side by side. Joan was only eleven when Sonny gave her a plastic friendship ring she would cherish as a keepsake among her most valuable possessions. She parted with it only when she felt that her granddaughter Allysyn, who was going through hard times in her teens, was in greater need of its special powers than she was.

This was a couple who, after their respective cancer diagnoses left them no hope for recovery, kept expressing thankfulness for going through end of life together. It was fitting that they entered the hospice program within months of each other and received care together in their home. They accepted that their time had come and developed small rituals of love surrounding their respective illnesses' symptom management. They would meet after midnight in the kitchen to take their pills and share a cookie. Their daughter Lisa would often find them there at the kitchen table, chattering and laughing like a pair of teenagers in love. They slept in side-by-side recliners, holding hands. When they were finally bedridden, they fell asleep, still holding hands over the railings of the hospital beds that Lisa, a nurse, had ordered for her home.

Despite the severity of his condition, Sonny never complained about the pain from his cancer or the rheumatoid arthritis that was crippling him. He showed concern only for his soulmate. When the suffering became so excruciating that his treatments had to be stopped, his only wish was that he go first because he could not imagine life without her.

Eventually, Sonny suffered symptoms that required him to be transferred from their home to the Hospice Inpatient Unit. They were both weakened yet interdependent and neither was able to function without the other, so Joan was transferred to the inpatient unit along with him. Against protocol, both husband and wife were placed in a single room with adjoining beds, which allowed them to still hold hands.

Joan and Sonny's anniversary was sacred to them. The date was approaching in a few short days following Sonny's admission to the Hospice Inpatient Unit, and Joan was anxious that they celebrate one last time. She was particularly insistent about this wish, and as usual, Sonny listened. On their anniversary, June 3, 2016, friends and family gathered at the hospice to celebrate. The staff joined them.

After the celebrations were over, Joan asked to be left alone with her husband. When her daughter returned to the room, Joan was crying. She confessed to Lisa that she had told Sonny, "It is okay to go now."

Within twenty-four hours, Sonny died, in peace, fifty-seven years to the day after he vowed to honor, love, and cherish his bride "till death do us part."

But this is not where Joan and Sonny's story ends. After Sonny's passing, Joan's health began to deteriorate rapidly, and her subsequent end-of-life experiences and visions helped her, as well as her family, cope with the deep wound left by Sonny's loss. When Joan returned from the Hospice Inpatient Unit, her dreams kept Sonny alive. During many nights, Lisa and her family could hear Joan calling out to her husband: "Come get me. I miss you! Sonny, come and get me!" The strength of these dreams would soon carry her from sleep to wakefulness, and Joan, fully lucid, would often claim to see Sonny in the room.

Joan and Sonny's story exemplifies the uniqueness and intensity with which end-of-life dreams and visions are experienced as a site of togetherness. Joan lived for two months beyond Sonny's death but never without him. She would call out to him every night and have visions of him every day.

Like Joan, eighty-nine-year-old Beverly experienced predeath dreams that took her back to her husband, her "accomplice" of forty-nine years. She was twenty years old when she first noticed the handsome and dapper Scottish immigrant who would sweep her off her feet. It was love at first sight, and Beverly and Bill were married less than a year later. Her husband had a contagious taste for music and dance, and they were soon sharing a passion for ballroom dancing that lasted for the remainder of their married life. Beverly's daughter, Susan, recalled with pride that her parents were so riveting as a couple that crowds at dance competitions would part to watch them do their glide. Through dance, her parents re-created, albeit in flashier outfits, the world of close partnership and loving complicity that defined their home life.

At life's end, Beverly's dreams would take her back to the protected space on the dance floor, where Bill and she had excelled as a team. She saw herself in close embrace with her soulmate, moving to the enrapturing beat of the music. Even the act of recounting this dream made Beverly look blissful. I still smile at the thought of the unassuming mother and secretary by day owning the highly stylized and theatrical form of ballroom dancing by night. This was the stuff dreams are made of, the kind of transformation and secret life people look for in movies.

Still, the full meaning of Beverly's dreams and visions would have eluded me had Susan not shared another pertinent detail about her mother's past. Beverly's own mother had been overly demanding, and she had mocked her daughter for being heavy and having "two left feet." In light of this history of shaming, it became obvious that Beverly's dreams of dancing were also about righting this wrong. The once chubby and clumsy girl had turned into an elegant and confident woman who, in her own words, "felt like a princess in Bill's arms." The world of dance not only brought into view the love she shared with her partner, but also symbolized the restitution of the self-love and -esteem eroded by her mother's humiliating comments. As with Patricia's crosswords visions, Beverly's dreams of dancing were about a shared love that served as a catalyst for self-confidence and harmony. Love is at its best when loving the other enables and overlaps with the ability to love together. Both Patricia's and Beverly's end-of-life experiences put them back in touch with that kind of true love, the one that embodies the best of all worlds.

Beverly's beloved Bill died at the young age of sixty-eight. For the rest of her widowed life, Beverly protested that she felt "robbed." But now, as she lay dying, the emptiness she had felt for two decades was finally filled with familiar love. Her feelings of loneliness were giving way to those of a hopeful reunion. Her pre-death dreams reconnected her with the strongest source of attachment and support she had known.

The ripple effect of her end-of-life experiences did not stop there. My old friend Patricia fittingly called it "the drop that ripples out into a pond." Sometimes it is a child, sometimes a parent whose love emboldens one to look outside oneself to what matters and resonates for others. End-of-life experiences embody the connectivity between and across lives. The love that the dreams and visions of our patients make visible is one that grows beyond those through whom it came to be, and extends from the dreamworld into waking reality and back again.

Love may be something that initially happens between two people, but it never rests there. It trickles into other lives and generations, and does not stop at the living. It is also won through hundreds of daily acts of mutual care, selfless gestures of affection, and words of concern whose cumulative force makes us who we are, over the thousands of days that constitute a shared lifetime.

For Susan, the love that she felt for her mother brought her parents full circle. After the terminal diagnosis Beverly had received a year earlier, she began receiving hospice care at her daughter's home, and the closeness the two women would share during those final months was one of the most obvious legacies of Beverly and Bill's love story, one that was all the more meaningful to her because the vital mother-daughter connection she shared was not biological.

When Bill and Beverly discovered they could not have children, they decided to adopt. They arrived at the Catholic Charities orphanage in Cleveland, where they lived at the time. They were full of indescribable anticipation and joy, but were also wondering how one decides on the child who will carry one's hopes and wishes into the future. As is human nature, the awaiting parents were drawn to the one whose eyes were bright with life, cheeks rosy and full, a healthy and active baby boy. They were screened as an adoptive couple, approved, and several weeks later, they left the orphanage with the chubby-cheeked, smiling infant who would grow up to be Susan's brother, Scott.

Beverly was thrilled at the prospect of raising this much-wanted child, but over time, she remained haunted by those whose eyes had not drawn her in, the sick and rejected. She felt guilty for having chosen based on traits over which no child has power. She and Bill had room for one more in their lives and hearts, and by the time Scott was three, they went back to the orphanage with a different agenda—to choose the sickest baby in the ward, the child most in need of their love. This was Susan.

Susan had been born to a seventeen-year-old girl, a rape survivor who had tried to induce an abortion by starving herself. As a result, Susan was born prematurely, with a host of medical issues that required two abdominal surgeries before she turned nine months old. She had been in several foster home placements, but no one had wanted to keep the medically complex child.

Susan remembers to this day her dying mother's account of the adoption. I was also privileged to have been present when Beverly recalled telling her husband, "Let's take the one in the back with the vacant eyes. She needs us." She then paused and, pointing to Susan, added, "And now I need her." I was touched by the simplicity with which she recognized the role reversal in this story of interdependence like it was the most natural thing in the world. And it was.

Susan proceeded to pull out pictures, taken of the family shortly after the adoption. In a particularly revealing one, Beverly is holding a mischievous-looking three-year-old Scott wearing a cowboy hat, and an affectless Susan, whose blank stare is at odds with the warmth of her mother's embrace. As she showed me the picture, Susan remarked that she had received so much love that she was unaware of any negative effects left by her early trauma and abandonment. She had always thought of herself as "the luckiest daughter in the world."

As Susan described the circuitous route through which she came to receive the gift of family, I took stock of the arbitrary but also serendipitous way in which life can take the most momentous turn. It was fate that placed Susan and her brother on Beverly and Bill's path at the right time and in the right place. It was also fate and history that set in motion the events of 1942 that led a boy in war-torn Poland to grab a girl by the hand and save her.

The proverbial full circle also defined Beverly's story: she would die in the loving care of the once sickly child she had taken in. Her selfless act was returned to her in the love and care she received at life's close, and that gave her the protected space she needed to fully experience her dreams and visions.

End-of-life experiences offer a blueprint for the workings of the love they catalyze, stage, and restore. They epitomize attachments that do not stop at the living—or the dead, for that matter. It is this infinite process of human interconnectivity that end-of-life experiences crystalize, the awareness that love's scope is never restricted to those who feel and enact it, nor does it know of expiration dates.

As Joan and Sonny's daughter Lisa once remarked, her mother's end-of-life experiences kept Sonny's love alive as much for herself as for her grieving family. In fact, it was only after Joan died that Lisa finally grieved her father. The daughter's sense of loss was triggered not by her dad's actual death but by the passing of her mother, who was no longer there to keep his memory alive. Still, long after both Sonny and Joan had passed, it was the lingering effects of Joan's pre-death experiences that helped carry the family through the grieving process. Knowing that her parents had never really been separated in life or in death helped Lisa cope with her own feelings of loss.

---

Like Lisa, Benny's daughter Maureen knows something about the shared cumulative love of nurturing, partnering, caring for, and grieving. She too has been a serial caregiver, for several years now—for her in-laws; for her dying mother, Gloria, three years earlier; and finally for her heartbroken father.

I remember visiting Benny after he had moved in with his daughter and son-in-law. "Benny is asleep," Maureen told me upon opening the door, as if to apologize. I was touched by the warmth and friendliness of the surroundings. She had obviously rearranged the furniture in her living space to accommodate her dad's needs. I had seen this before. Living rooms or family rooms are often completely transformed for the sake of a dying family member's ease of function and comfort—decor and design sacrificed for the sake of functionality. Sometimes, the furniture is pushed to the edges of rooms for wheelchair access. The living room may become cluttered with favorite belongings or one too many mismatched couches. Or, as with Joan and Sonny, a hospital bed or two would appear in the center of the family room, strategically angled in relation to the television set.

For Maureen, rearranging her living space also meant scattering pictures of Benny's earlier life all over the room. It was a genuine gallery of framed memories from the late 1940s and '50s, adorning every flat surface available. The pictures were mostly of Benny's wife, Gloria, smiling at her First Communion, their wedding, the baptism of their first child, in the customary family portraits reproduced in various poses over time. These were Benny's memories, not Maureen's. Her wedding picture was hanging on the wall behind her father's chair, outside his field of vision, and displaying the vibrant colors and modern outfits of a later generation.

There is a role reversal that occurs when caring for elderly parents who become more childlike at life's end. The process demands that as caregivers we not only adopt the position of the parent vis-à-vis our dying relative but also that we center them. Maureen knew that better than anyone. She knew that her father's cognitive abilities were compromised by disease and frailty. Gone were the days he could form new memories and have new experiences on which to draw. What was left instead were decades-old memories and end-of-life experiences in which he felt alive. He might not remember what he ate for breakfast, but he could recall the color of the dress his wife had worn when they met. He may not function cognitively in the present, but he remained alive in the past, and his sense of self was increasingly more familiar with the then than the now. It was a time capsule of sorts, which placed him in an era with which he was most familiar, and where only long-past memories were accessible to his recall.

This is why Maureen surrounded her father with pictures and furniture from his previous life. They grounded him. By postdating everything, she could re-create the only reality that still centered him, that of his youth and marriage. She had facilitated a time travel not only to contextualize his surroundings but also to allow him to relive what was still familiar. She knew she had done right by him when one day she saw him pick up one of her mother's photographs and talk to it as if Glo was right there, ready to answer. Maureen had helped her father return to a time and place in which he was more than just a dying man.

For Maureen, the protected space of caretaking was also an occasion for her to find and center herself. She was grateful to have gotten to know her father better, this man "who believed in giving many chances, in loving life, working hard, and treating people with kindness." She could reacquaint herself with his past, reputation, and legendary decency. At the same time, caring for Benny had involved reassessing her own sense of values. It had grounded her in the knowledge of love's continuity as well as in the importance of the daily tasks and routines she had so expertly managed for his care. She proudly shared that although his doctors had given him at most six months to live, the date had come and gone. That was three years ago.

Some people are so used to the fabric of love with which their family structure is woven that they seem unaware of the exceptional quality of the bonds that shape their lives. It takes another's gaze to reveal the extraordinary at the heart of the ordinary, and the warmth of a heart that is carved in snow. End-of-life experiences also provide an opportunity to recognize the possibility of grace when, as Patricia put it, "the now becomes the end," because they provide a context for lifelong love stories that stretch into eternity and back.

At its most meaningful, life is about this "tiny little thing" we feel for those we love—mother, father, child, spouse, or pet—and the love we get back. It may have been eighty years ago or twenty years since that love was expressed, but how our mother said good-bye or how our father waited for us each day after school matters in ways we seldom register when these events occur. End-of-life experiences highlight the moments in our past that mattered but may have been taken for granted, what happened when we were too busy making other plans. They help reframe dying in a way that is not about last words and lost love but about strengthened selves and unbreakable bonds between and across lives. Joan, Beverly, Patricia, and Benny were not merely widowed elders in the twilight of life, but actualized human beings with inner lives full of love, loyalty, and connection. Their pre-death dreams took them beyond physical frailty to a place where love is perennial and "attempts things beyond its strength."

# the child's language of death

The Child's faith is new—
Whole—like His Principle—
Wide—like the Sunrise
On fresh Eyes—
Never had a Doubt—

—EMILY DICKINSON

When I met Jessica, she was thirteen, and I didn't know how to help a child die. And truth be told, I had never wanted to learn. It was the horrible incongruity of a child in hospice care, the cruel absurdity of life ending at its beginning, and my strong aversion to pediatrics. Children in distress had always unhinged me in a way that made me feel less capable as a doctor. The feeling was compounded by my being the father of two young girls.

So when the time came to meet Jessica face-to-face, I did not think that I was the right person for the task, let alone the right doctor. Jessica had Ewing sarcoma, a rare and malignant form of bone-based cancer. It had been three years since her diagnosis, and she was my first "pediatric hospice patient." That is the phrase doctors use to mitigate the unimaginable reality of a child dying.

I knew that my reaction would be visceral, so much so that I worried that any medical expertise I may offer could not compensate for my fears. And I was right. It didn't. It didn't need to. As I walked into her room, trying to be the doctor I thought she needed me to be, I quickly realized that no level of medical expertise would be a match for her innocent wisdom.

I was bracing myself for an excruciating conversation. Instead, I encountered a bright-eyed young girl who was eager to chat about her day, her mom, her pets, and her dreams. Jessica did not pause to mourn the life she would not get to live or to talk about the career or kids she would not have. She had no regrets to mull over, or could-have-beens, missed opportunities, or any of the considerations that often darken adult consciousness. She was too busy living in the now, the same spunky and affectionate little girl her mom had always known, notwithstanding her painful symptoms and the treatment's side effects. She was too enchanted by the heavenly world she saw in her dreams, where her recently deceased dog, Shadow, was roaming free and healthy again. She was too focused on getting to ninth grade, her personal goal. She still wanted to be a kid doing what kids do. If she talked about death, it was incidental.

But it also went deeper than that.

Children have few reference points for death; they lack a language for mortality, let alone for "battling" it. In fact, the war metaphor so commonly used to describe living with a terminal illness could not be any less appropriate than in relation to a child's experience of dying. Children don't fight death. They live every moment not as though it is their last but as if it is going to last. Acceptance is not a state they have to work to achieve. They inhabit and embody it all at the same time.

Neither Jess nor her mother, Kristin, were given a prognosis or survival rate at the time of diagnosis, and they didn't ask. Jessica was dying—which is to say living, fully aware of her impending death—but no one had ever explicitly told her. She just knew. Children have an intuitive ability to understand when death is imminent. Denial is as foreign to them as it is natural in adults. So, like most dying children, Jessica understood more than she told, or was told. It was the show-not-tell of her dreams and visions that informed her. She dreamed in distinct tones and textures, which not only created awareness of her impending death but also secured her in love.

Children's end-of-life experiences, like those of other patients, feature loved ones who come back to them. Unlike adults, however, children often do not know someone who has already died. As a result, the deceased who have loved them best and come back to them in the end are often beloved pets. It was visions of her dog, Shadow, as well as of her mom's deceased friend Mary that populated Jess's dreams and visions as her time drew closer.

Unlike adults, who think of animals in terms of their shorter life-span, children see pets as lifetime companions. Often the family pet arrives before the child is born and is therefore intrinsic to the family and their world. The human-animal distinction does not resonate in their consciousness—or in their unconscious, for that matter. Their relationship with domestic animals is often how they learn to engage with others, nurture, and love, and how they encounter mortality for the very first time. Jessica's description of her dog best illustrates how, for her, he was family: "We were close, even though I didn't like him half the time because he would always be on my butt, but I still loved him." Shadow was an indolent, begging, and often annoying seventy-pound black Labrador mix that had been, along with her mother, her rock.

Etched in my mind is the memory of this composed, strong-willed girl, sitting cross-legged on the couch, hands on her lap, matter-of-factly answering my questions. "My dreams that I have are good dreams now," Jessica would explain in her disarmingly direct way. She never veered from this straightforward form of expression, not even when a camera crew showed up to film an interaction for a documentary. By then, my questions were somewhat predictable—I always asked about her health, daily routines, sleep, and state of mind. All the same, Jess sat there like a Zen master, gracing me with her undivided attention. She then articulated her careful and thoughtful answers to each question. "I dream of my old dog Shadow that passed away. He is in a good place; he is running, having fun but then runs away and I never see him again. I feel like it is his way of saying good-bye. He occasionally comes to see me, and I have a feeling he is there to say it is okay, I am in a safe place."

Jessica was quick to make sense of Shadow's return in her

dream as "the meaning of love." He was a scout, not a pallbearer, and he had come back to bring her the love and support she needed to embark on her end-of-life journey. The difficult conversation about dying I had once dreaded had become completely irrelevant. She had actually been having it all along with herself, in her end-of-life dreams, and these had already provided her with all the answers she was either seeking or needing.

Before Jessica, I assumed that for a child to understand death, I would need to paint her a picture. I remember strategizing about using simple language and imagery, as well as age-appropriate references. But my presumption was a function of a misplaced condescension, not of the reality of a child's dying experience.

I was stunned to find out that this child had a better understanding of her own mortality than I could ever have imagined. What adults first experience as grief, Jessica had already reframed into sensory images of joy, color, warmth, and security; what we perceive as separation, she was experiencing as a loving reunion under Shadow's guidance. Her dog's return in dreams signaled that the end was close, but it did not trigger any fear of the unknown. Instead, it brought about solace and the comfort of knowing that she would be entering sheltering, safe, and familiar territory alongside a furry friend. A child's death may be unimaginable to adults, but it is fodder for the grace of the imagination to kids.

Like most dying children, Jessica did not mark a clear distinction between her immediate world and the imaginary one of her dreams. Rather, she lived her recurring dreams as if they were actual visions. In fact, she could not always tell which was which. "Usually, I just lie there on my back and try to reenact that dream. And I think about what just happened to wake me up but I do get afraid because I see how dark my room is. One night there was one long black thing there—that was Shadow by my bed. I went down to the ground [to pet him] and it looked like his head went up, and then it was gone." What she saw felt so real that she would reach out to touch it.

I remember trying to put her experience into words for her. I described it as a dream blending into her reality when she opened her eyes. She looked at me, puzzled, as if unconvinced. My language still implied a separation between sleeping and waking, and as such, it failed to resonate with the lived experience of her dream. When I asked her if Shadow ever spoke to her, she gave me the "Duh!" eye roll of a teenager and answered, "Dogs don't talk." For Jessica, the blurring of the line between reality and her dreamworld entailed no lapse in logic or in her reasoning abilities.

Over time, I learned my lesson, which was to say less. Instead, I sat in awe as Jessica shared perceptions and experiences that contained an understanding of a disease progression for which I had no words.

She went on to dream about Mary, her mother's best friend who'd died at age thirty-five, when Jessica was only eight: "Mary is one of my mom's best friends who passed away from leukemia. I think I was pretty close to her, and she was very close to my mom. I liked her. She was very nice. I'd seen her in my mom's room. Coming up the stairs, I was going into my room and stopped when I saw from the corner of my eye someone playing with my mom's curtains. She had her favorite shirt on. My mom told me that it was, because I told my mom it was a gray-and-blue checkered flannel shirt." I was somewhat surprised by her dreaming self's stoicism in the presence of a dead person walking. I asked if her mom was there. "Yes, she was. Mary didn't look at me; I had a feeling if I called out her name she would look at me, but I didn't want to scare my mom." Jessica was the only child of a single mother, which left her with one last uncertainty once her concern about dying was resolved: "What will I do without my mom?" The vision of this mother surrogate, her mother's best friend, in her mother's room, brought tremendous peace to her. She felt "relief and happiness." She continued, "Mary was a very strong person, and I know that I am strong and my mom tells me all the time that I am like her."

Kristin, who never left her daughter's side, reminded her, "You told me all the time that 'Mom, I saw an angel,' and then you were able to go to sleep."

"Yes." Jessica nodded. "I was able to go to sleep. It was really comforting, and I was not afraid of it at all."

Jessica was at first reluctant to share her vision of Mary with Kristin for fear of unsettling or frightening her mother. This remarkable selflessness at the time of death is a common theme among dying children. I have yet to meet many children who leave this world without trying to spare or protect those who are left behind.

Jessica's dreams had staged a two-act play that both embodied and solved the puzzle her death would otherwise have been for her. First, her dog "came back to me and it means that I am okay, and I am not alone." Then, a new concern emerged from the recognition of impending death, namely how she was going to live without her mom. Jessica did not know of a world or a self that did not include her mother. Their relationship was truly symbiotic, and it had only become more so through illness. Jessica's dependence on her mother defined her sense of self, so much so that what her soul feared most was an existence without her. This was the source of a deep anxiety she could not fully articulate but that her second dream of Mary addressed and resolved all the same.

As adults, we often assume that acceptance at life's end is about accepting one's death. In keeping with this assumption, many think that my job as a palliative care doctor is to guide dying patients to that point, to help them come to terms with the idea of their finality. But that is not always the case. The knowledge of death is never the end of the discussion in hospice care; it is its beginning. We ask questions such as "How do you feel?"; "Are you going to be okay?"; "Are you at peace?" not just because the answer matters but because the process does. And patients' end-of-life dreams play a big role in this progression. They are not the end or the goal. They are the tools we use even if, or rather precisely because, they are not of our own making.

Until Jessica, I could not imagine that children would have access to their own set of tools during the dying process. I assumed that a young mind was not fit to handle a conversation about life's end, and I failed to appreciate the sophisticated ways in which it may have occurred. Jessica had an understanding of death that exceeded anything I could have imagined; she created connections, abstractions, and conclusions I could not have given her, and they required no words or comments. All I had to do was listen.

A child's innocence goes infinitely deeper than ignorance. Unbeknownst to her, Jessica's end-of-life experiences were teaching her, as well as her caretakers, how to cope with the inconceivable. Most importantly, for Kristin, they helped initiate the process she could not have consciously accepted, that of letting go. But it was not of her daughter that Kristin was letting go—she could never do that—it was of denial.

Mother and daughter shared an unspoken language and a spiritual bond that have carried over to this day. Six years after her daughter's death, Kristin still feels Jessica's presence. She still decorates her house for every holiday because "Jess would not have it any other way." She still cares for her little girl's spoiled and overweight orange cat, Lulu, who continues to wear the silly ornament Jess once attached to her collar. She still remembers what Jess wore on Monday, September 13, 2010, the day they received the devastating diagnosis. And she smiles at the memories accumulated during the precious two years, six months, and four days she still had with her daughter.

Kristin may have let go, but she has not moved on. She doesn't need to. No parent ever does. Acceptance does not require or justify it. There is nothing broken in our relationship to our children from which we would need to distance ourselves in death. There is nothing with which to replace or supplant it. For Kristin especially, there was no moving on beyond the legacy of strength and magnanimity Jess had left behind, only moving *with*. Years later, when I met Kristin to reminisce about her formidable little girl, she could not help but wonder at her own inexplicable strength and ability to speak at her daughter's memorial, so shortly after her baby girl's passing. "What mother does that?" she exclaimed. "Jess's," I answered without hesitation.

It is often our kids who make us into the parents we didn't know we could be.

This is also true of Michele, another warrior mom who didn't know how strong she was until called upon by the needs of her ill child. The war metaphor, as inappropriate as it may be in reference to those living with a terminal disease, has profound resonance when it comes to the parents of dying children. I have known parents who, in the midst of unimaginable sorrow, found in themselves the courage to help their child live as full a life as possible in the space that separates dying from death. I have seen them confront a medical system that loses its way transitioning from *whether* a patient dies to *how*. I have watched such parents' persistence in a downhill battle whose successes are measured in smiles and milestones, not victories.

When I first met Virginia Rose, aka Ginny, she looked half her age. Stunted growth was only one of the side effects of the whole brain radiation therapy she had received ten years prior to treat her original illness, leukemia. The other unintended consequence was the brain tumor that would first be mistakenly diagnosed as a slow-growing, low-grade form of cancer. She was fourteen and a half years old, and her family had been getting ready to celebrate the tenth anniversary of her being cured from leukemia.

With the courage that had always defined her, Michele, Ginny's mother, braced herself for another protracted battle against a second cancer diagnosis. Within months, she realized that her child was declining faster than she expected, and she could not grasp what was happening. It was unclear to her whether Ginny's worsening neurological condition was due to her illness or its treatment, or which symptoms were permanent and which were reversible. She did not know if this was what the disease with the unpronounceable name was supposed to look like. Michele did not know—did not really *want* to know—if her child was dying. Her mother's instinct had so much as told her, but no one had actually clarified things for her. She remained confused as to the when and the how. She was lost on a journey without a map, grieving while confused by the spiral of modern medicine, which failed to provide the open and direct communication she needed most.

Eventually, Michele took her weakening daughter to the hospital and put her stake in the ground: "I am not leaving until someone tells me what is going on with my kid." She was one of many parents I have known who, suffering with the pain of uncertainty, have taken their dying child to the ER in search of answers rather than intervention. It is not the truth these parents can't face; it is the lack of guidance and direction they find unbearable.

On the fateful day Michele took Ginny in, her right to inquire and question on behalf of her child was met with resentment by the covering physician. Uncertain of all the diagnostic implications, she pressed so hard that the exasperated doctor threw three medical papers down at her in lieu of the compassionate conversation she was craving and deserved. She picked up the documents and fumbled her way through medical jargon to discover the devastating truth no parent should ever have to face alone: Ginny had a different type of brain tumor than doctors had initially diagnosed—a glioblastoma, an incurable form of brain cancer. Although pathology can be confusing and there are many subtleties within diagnoses, the implications of the second one were life-altering. The nomenclature may be irrelevant, but Michele had been working on the premise that her daughter was suffering from a potentially manageable condition, only to find out that her disease was terminal.

Health care often resembles an assembly line of highly technological and specialized medical interventions whose fragmented workings can leave grieving families guessing. As the surgeon and writer Atul Gawande puts it in his book *Being Mortal*, "Medical science has rendered obsolete centuries of experience, tradition, and language about our mortality and created a new difficulty for mankind: how to die." Health care today is doled out in installments that do not add up to a human story. Bodily organs get treated one part at a time, while the patient's humanity is often ignored. Medicine's best armature often fails to take the time to help parents understand what is happening to their dying child, how to help ease their child's final moments, or even how to recognize those moments.

In the time that had separated Ginny's two diagnoses, the hope-bearing one and the soul-crushing one, she had undergone several brain surgeries. These led to an increasing loss of neurological function, including complete paralysis on the left side of her body. She also developed a postoperative infection of her skull that simply refused to heal. Because her immune system was compromised, multiple rounds of antibiotics failed to stop the infection from spreading to the overlying scalp.

The Ginny who suffered from these grueling symptoms, the one I had read about in my medical notes, was not the Ginny I met and got to know. Michele's Ginny, the Ginny we remember and love, was not defined by the cancer and infection her body could not fight or the wheelchair she sat in. The Ginny we still smile and cry about was the young girl who, despite her disease complications, a drooping face, and an infected head wound, had retained a child's sense of wonder; the Ginny who remained, in Michele's words, "stubborn about wanting to learn," notwithstanding her impaired cognitive abilities, another side effect of whole brain radiation. It was the Ginny who, like any teen her age, enjoyed keeping abreast of the popular songs and artists of the day, the teen idols and entertainment news. It was the Ginny whose colorful head bandannas transformed the swelling wound that was her daily lot into a fashion statement of sorts; and the Ginny who, when asked if there was anything about her condition I should know, offered her most radiant grin before responding, simply and unaffectedly, "Yes, that I am beautiful."

I remember the cozy suburban house where Ginny lived with her mom, stepdad, and siblings. Everything about her living space spelled typical American teenager—except for the hospital bed, the metal hospital tray holding her medications, and the porta-pot in the corner of her room. She had an aquarium with two pet fish and owned every single sea-life plush animal toy from the Disney movie *Finding Nemo*. Her bedroom walls were covered with posters of the boy band One Direction. She delighted in singing the hits of her generation's teen heartthrobs and was especially partial to Justin Bieber and Shawn Mendes. I teased her about her fondness for Canadians. She smiled because she knew I was one too.

Ginny told me about the shadows she'd sometimes see flitting around her when she woke up at night. They used to frighten her, but after one particular dream experience, she started finding them comforting. The shift occurred during an MRI when she fell asleep inside the pulsing machine and had a vision of her beloved aunt Mimi, who had recently died. Like Jessica, Ginny did not have a complex vocabulary for dying, so she imagined a new reality based on the language and imagery she had at hand. In her dream, she saw her aunt in a castle "with a baby in the window, and you can see the sun through it." She could not have summoned a more beautiful and necessary metaphor for a rebirth in a world free from harm. There was warmth and light, in a structure that suggests both fortification and unrestricted protection. Ginny described her castle as "a safe place" for Aunt Mimi as well as for Grandma Rose, who had also died not long ago. Ginny could feel Mimi hugging her and whispering in her ear, "You've got to go back down there and fight."

Ginny had loved swimming when she was cancer-free, so her castle also had a pool. It set that stage for the activity that had brought her joy when she was healthy. Ginny also filled her dreams with a menagerie of the animals she had known, loved, and lost. Dogs, cats, and birds took turns appearing, resurrected as healthy versions of their living selves. When she woke up after the MRI, she was almost euphoric and proclaimed to her mother, "I'm going to be okay; I'm not alone."

Both Ginny and Jess created inner worlds that provided what their actual world could not—the opportunity to be made whole again. The presence of deceased animals brought back to life served as harbingers of health regained and made them feel safe, at ease, and loved.

Ginny, like Jess, already knew that she would be leaving the reality of the living and going to a place populated with the dead. Her dreams told her as much. As her disease progressed, her dreams multiplied, and so did the deceased animals and pets who were now enjoying health and freedom in "the castle." In this alternative world, the knowledge of impending death was integrated within the certainty of love from another existence, one freed from disease, just like the vision of her pets, whose unconditional love and acceptance she was also summoning. Ginny had no need for adult words, though she must have known that we did, because she provided them to us indirectly, through the songs she loved.

When I asked about her favorite music, Ginny would mention titles, and I would quickly expose my ignorance about her generation's musical tastes. She would graciously move on. It was a year and a half after her passing that I stopped to listen to the lyrics of one of her favorite songs, "Stitches" by Shawn Mendes, a song about the emotional wounds inflicted by unrequited love. Ginny knew all the words to this song. As my mind began to register what the words actually meant, I realized that to Ginny, there could not have been anything metaphorical about the physical and medical terms used by Mendes:

> I thought that I've been hurt before,
> but no one's ever left me quite this sore . . .
> Now I need someone to breathe me back to life,
> Got a feeling that I'm going under . . .
> I'll be needing stitches
> I'm tripping over myself
> Aching, begging you to come help

The refrain was even more heartbreaking:

Needle and the thread
Gotta get you out of my head
Needle and the thread
Gonna wind up dead

I was speechless. Yet again, I had made assumptions about the rudiments of a child's thought process, only to realize my limited understanding of it. At sixteen years old, Ginny was caught between childhood and adulthood, so the language through which she processed mortality belonged to both realms. She dreamt of heavenly castles while singing about real pain. She still wished for a time when stitches were enough to heal a wound.

Michele had never talked to Ginny about dying. She didn't need to. Six weeks before her death, Ginny texted her mom from her bedroom to say, "I wanna die. I am never gonna get better." She was fully cognizant of what her mother was trying so hard to repress. She also processed the truth in more than one script. Sometimes it was screens, songs, or dreams that conspired to make the unimaginable palatable, whether it was for the adults who couldn't accept it or for she herself, who already had.

In the days approaching her death, Ginny called out to her mother every fifteen minutes or so. One day, Michele had just returned to the kitchen, where she kept the transmitter unit of the baby monitor that was always in her daughter's room. She suddenly heard Ginny in animated conversation. She went back to her daughter's room to ask who she had been talking to. "I was talking to God," Ginny replied. "He's old, but he's kinda cute." And remarkably for a child who had not been raised with religion or going to church, she added, as if to reassure her mother, "I'm not going to be sick, you know, where I'm going. You know, to the castle."

After her encounter with God, Ginny stopped her pattern of repeatedly calling out to her mom. Her source of comfort had shifted to her rich inner world, one whose content she had once shared but no longer needed to. I saw Ginny the next day, and she was quiet and comfortable. She died four days later.

I think of Ginny often, but at no time did her memory haunt me more than when I met Sandra, a sixteen-year-old Syrian girl who had recently moved to the United States with her family.

This was a young girl whose parents had applied for refugee status thirteen years earlier. Now, less than six months after their arriving in their much-awaited new home, their only daughter had been transferred to the Hospice Inpatient Unit with widely metastatic bone cancer. Marine and Hanna, Sandra's mother and father, had hoped, against all odds, that relocating to the United States would help save their little girl. Deeply religious, they had seen the timing of their immigration to the most medically advanced country in the world as an answer to their prayers.

Sandra was sent to Hospice Buffalo from Roswell Park Comprehensive Cancer Center for management of her unrelenting pain. Her physical suffering, as well as the underlying disease, had escalated abruptly and, given her severe level of distress, home care would not have been appropriate.

At Hospice Buffalo, Sandra, desperate for relief, kept asking for "more pain medicine." I was stunned by the advanced stage of her disease and the ineffectiveness of her previous pain management, something I unfortunately witness too often in end-of-life care, especially for children for whom there is a greater reluctance to medicate.

Like many patients who experience severe suffering, Sandra had been left traumatized by her pain, in a manner not unlike PTSD. In a state of heightened fear, she now anticipated pain with any and all movement. She had understandably lost confidence in medicine's obligation to relieve suffering. Even so, Sandra expressed nothing but gratitude for the care she was receiving in this foreign land she would never get to call home.

When her family was out of earshot, Sandra requested full sedation. She confessed that she wanted to spare her mother and father the sight of her suffering, so she requested medicine "so I can just sleep." She was exhausted from her disease and struggled to remain alert and engaged, yet lessening the suffering of others meant more to her than letting go of her waning moments of wakefulness.

We developed a plan for managing Sandra's pain. The administered medication was effective and made her comfortable. She went from requesting to be made unconscious to asking to stay at Hospice Buffalo: "I don't want to go home."

Unlike her parents, Sandra spoke fluent English. Given how much she had suffered, her priority was to remain where she found comfort. Home was where pain was, where it was insurmountable, where she had hurt more than she could love.

That is how I first realized that she knew.

She knew, even though her parents were doing everything in

their power to keep the truth from her. They did not want her to think that she was dying. As profoundly Catholic as they were, they even declined the offer of a chaplain to be present at her bedside. That may have inadvertently given her a clue as to her condition. There would be no conversation, spiritual advising, or coming to terms for their little girl. They wanted their vibrant daughter to continue believing in treatments, in the possibility of a cure, in miracles. I intuitively understood where this insistence came from. Sandra was a fighter, a force of nature, and seeing her resigned to her tragic fate would have meant losing her twice. They could not deprive her of hope without renouncing theirs. It was too much to ask of parents who had sacrificed everything to give their daughter a better life she would never get to live.

Mom and Dad kept taking turns at Sandra's bedside while Tony and Remi, their family friends, came as often as they could to serve as interpreters. Tony and Remi were the friends who had provided the Haddad family a home upon their arrival in the United States, and Sandra was like a daughter to them. They spoke of her with as much pride as if they were her parents. And her brothers concurred, in a loving stereo, that she was smarter than both of them combined.

I never felt comfortable with my inability to communicate directly with the family, but I appreciated their willingness to interpret for me. I also knew that not everything required interpretation. What needed no translation, for instance, was the tragedy of this young girl and her family, or the love that emanated from parent to child, brother to sister, and that, as weak as she was, Sandra reflected back to every single one of them.

As Sandra got relief from her pain, she once again more closely resembled the carefree young girl her friends and relatives had once known, whose vibrancy and selflessness were so intense that the world got noticeably darker when it lost her. This was the Sandra who, caught between two cultures and two languages, had danced and prayed her way into both; the Sandra who told me about the parties she had gone to in Syria and photos of which she could still access via social media; the Sandra who taught herself English in preparation for her emigration and who, when she landed in a cancer hospital, started teaching her nurses all the Arabic dance moves she knew. This was also the girl who, on her way back from treatment one day, would stand up in Tony's convertible, stretch out her arms, and scream with such joy that he too was transported to a time when reckless abandon trumped legalities; the girl who, when bedridden, would call out to Tony's wife, Remi, to come and play cards with her: "Remi, I took morphine . . . we can play"; the Sandra whose videos document this remarkable paradox—that of Sandra dancing, at every event, to any song, on benches, in hallways, in full view of crowds as well as in the privacy of her own home, despite her disabled arm, despite the bandanna and her unmistakable pallor.

Like Jess and like Ginny, Sandra was old enough to know, and far too young to die. And as with them, it was her recurring dreams that took care of revealing the truth we had been directed to hide. Sandra dreamed again and again that she was climbing the side of a mountain while people below were trying to drag her back down and prevent her from reaching the angels above. She could see a cross at the top of the mountain, which, when she finally reached it, made her feel pain-free. This was a recurring dream sequence that she shared often and with many. It was strikingly vivid, so much so that she got flustered in the telling. What bound her to earth came with extraordinary pain, and her dream, in enacting a release from it, staged the promise of a life relived without suffering. It helped her forge her own way outside of the medical care and spiritual guidance she was thankful for but that could not make her whole again. Through her end-of-life experiences, she created a world that helped her feel unmoored and unburdened, free from doubt and bodily harm.

Sandra came from a deeply devout culture, so it made sense that her end-of-life dreams and visions were contextualized within the symbolism of faith. Yet the story ending remained the same as for Jess and Ginny no matter how different the imagery or references. It was a similar tale of promise, health, and warmth, one so life-affirming that she was left feeling reconciled with the "will of God."

This was a story whose meaning required no explanation for most of us at the bedside. Upon hearing it, Tony, the family friend, immediately recognized what Sandra's parents could not face. In fact, he became so convinced of the imminence of her death that he was prompted to initiate, for her parents' sake, what they could not bring themselves to even think about, namely the funeral arrangements.

Unbeknownst to her family, Sandra had gone on to say her good-byes on Facebook a week before her death. She announced to her Syrian friends that this would be her last post "for a while." But what she left on her Facebook wall was nothing short of an elegy whose meaning will not get lost in translation: "It's true that I am still too young to talk about my life experience, but through my illness, I have a feeling that I gained a lot in terms of maturity. I learned that we should all do our best to spread joy even if we are in pain or unhappy. Don't think, plan, or work for the thereafter. Live day by day. Live in the moment. Because these moments won't return and because God's plan for you will happen regardless." Sandra did what most of us could not do. She said good-bye, and she did so on her own terms, in her own language, and in the medium of her time. In doing so, she shared the wisdom that she had accumulated in her short life and through her illness: the importance of faith, gratitude for every lived moment, and the responsibility to share joy.

It is because the idea of a dying child is so inconceivable that children's apparent serenity about death is so surprising. Yet it is as true for them as it is for adults that end-of-life dreams and experiences are full of the events and people and pets they need to be able to approach death with dignity and peace.

Those of us who were privileged to know Jessica, Ginny, and Sandra were left to struggle with a sense of meaningless loss when they died. Death in childhood is like an unfilled promise, and it is always a tragedy. Yet dying children move on without the doubts and regrets adults are left to harbor. Children don't share our despair and worldly pain. To put it simply, our fears are not theirs. They don't talk of their life ending as an experience cut short. Where we see loss, they see castles, angels, and loyal animals; they feel warmth and meet old friends; they hear music. Children find their own language that we cannot comprehend—an acceptance of mortality, a place where different forms of hope and release reside, and where unyielding love is a given.

At death's door, children leave us with lessons of resilience and grace. Yet for those of us left behind, empty and in pain, a child's death remains beyond our ability to comprehend. In these moments, we would do well to remember that children, unlike adults, experience end of life without getting mired in an endless search for meaning or forgiveness. As Emily Dickinson so beautifully wrote, "The child's faith is new," and they live their final days as though "they never had a doubt." They see "rainbows, as the common way." So perhaps it is best to let our sense of meaninglessness be tempered with reverence and awe for three young girls who found in their dreams what our shared reality could not provide: final peace.

# of different minds

Out beyond the ideas of wrongdoing and rightdoing,
there is a field.
I'll meet you there.

—RŪMĪ

The pages of this book are filled with an array of voices, from children and parents to spouses and siblings, from cops and criminals to the forgotten and the forlorn. Each reveals in his or her own way how, regardless of the lives led and experiences had, humanity's final moments do not merely consist of a passive disintegration of the flesh. Instead, life's end is about active and affirming inner processes, often with significant psychological and spiritual benefits for the dying. But what about people whose minds function differently? Those with cognitive or perceptual impairments, those categorized or labeled as mentally ill, demented, disabled, or "neuro-atypical," whose voices and stories are often hidden and marginalized in life? Do the labels and preconceptions that so often limit them in life also do so at the end, preventing them from partaking of the complex spiritual transformation this book has identified in others?

Experiences of dying and the opportunities for enrichment and fulfillment they offer are an aspect of our humanity that is even more overlooked when it comes to people with cognitive and developmental conditions. This is true whether the impairment is mild, as in Maggie's case, or more severe, as with advanced dementia.

Maggie was diagnosed with cerebral palsy in early childhood. Cerebral palsy is a neurological disorder caused by brain damage incurred either in utero or during birth. There is no cure, but the symptoms don't usually worsen with age, and Maggie led a long and fulfilled life with the knowledge that she was different and the certainty that she was loved. At seventy-five, she was admitted to our Hospice Inpatient Unit after opting to discontinue chemotherapy treatments for breast cancer, a decision that her husband of fifty years begrudged her. He wanted her to keep fighting, and she wanted to keep living, without the complications of the medical treatment she deemed futile. So she made her decision the same way she always did, without afterthought. Instead, while at Hospice Buffalo, she began revisiting her childhood memories of unadulterated family bliss and the "it takes a village" upbringing she had enjoyed while growing up in a working-class Buffalo neighborhood.

Maggie had been born to Dorothy and George, first-generation Polish immigrants, and she had been raised surrounded by love, music, tradition, joy, and laughter. Her story was inseparable from that of her immigrant community and their status as blue collar at a time when a lack of career options and financial means led to interdependence and mutual support.

Maggie grew up without the benefit of the Americans with Disabilities Act, without the enriched services or the widespread recognition that people with disabilities constitute a disenfranchised population. But this lack of policies, official practices, and procedures also meant that there was no classification or codification that would have separated her from others. Instead, she grew up feeling valued for who she was rather than defined by who she wasn't; she was given an identity and a sense of self-worth. Her life included challenges, such as a speech impediment and a learning disability, but was not limited by them. Regardless of her language skills or mode of delivery, her voice was cherished. Her difference was part of the rich tapestry that bound her to her close-knit community. This is also why Maggie's tale was predominantly one of happiness, not just within the confines of her home but whenever she walked down her street. Her "village" didn't reduce her to a label and recognized her humanity in its full complexity.

I have always been humbled by those who, born with challenges and in the absence of opportunity, embody happiness. Here sat Maggie, dying yet beaming a toothless smile, still playful, generous, and joyful; she was a mystery and a miracle rolled into one. She had succeeded in life by every true measure of success, through love given and received, and she knew it.

I had to ask: "How was it for you growing up with cerebral palsy?" Without missing a beat, Maggie told me about the "cheese bus," which was what schoolkids called the small bus that transported children with disabilities. Maggie was only twelve years old when she first refused to ride the cheese bus. She opted to walk forty-five minutes to and from school, in rain, sleet, and snow. She had grown up with a sense of belonging that was incompatible with anything that would mark her as indelibly different—the cheese bus was never an option. Walking was the price she was willing to pay for her dignity, and every step of the way was worth it to her.

Maggie didn't need or want to be the same as everyone else. She just wanted to preserve the gift she had been given in childhood—a sense of identity rooted in difference, not deficiency. At twelve, she was doing her part to create a world where differences are cause for celebration and where independence does not preclude interdependence.

Not surprisingly, Maggie's end-of-life experiences avoided the cheese bus as well. She had taken care of that thorny issue as a child. Instead, in her dreams, she got to relive one of the happiest moments of her childhood, the day in eighth grade when her classmates motioned for her to come to the classroom window. There, in the distance, she could see her grandfather playing the accordion and entertaining a large audience. People were clapping and dancing, while more kept joining in. For the young girl who had never won a prize, this was the biggest victory of them all: she was the grandchild of the kind and talented old man who entertained crowds both near and far. These were "her people," and she felt immense pride. This scene was the one she relived most frequently in her dreams, always deriving pleasure and a sense of wholeness from it—a reminder that she had always belonged and still mattered.

Maggie's pre-death experiences reflected not only how she

had lived, surrounded by family and community, but also the lightness and playfulness with which she moved through life. As a grown, married woman, Maggie had become known in her neighborhood as Grandma Moo Moo, mostly for her love of cows. This time, however, she embraced the new label. Her daughter Bernice recalled how the neighborhood children all "ran to Grandma Moo Moo as soon as they saw her," wanting hugs. Maggie kept "popsicles in the fridge" for them at all times and enjoyed being "a mom to all neighbors."

The cheerfulness that defined Maggie's life was mirrored in the humor with which she relayed her other dream's content. I remember when she began describing her recurring visions of a blanket moving across the room. It finally got snagged, exposing her deceased parents underneath. No matter how often Maggie shared this dream, it was always with sheer glee. Her reaction was partly due to her father's startled expression in the dream. He would raise his index finger to his mouth and murmur, "You are not supposed to see us," while reassuring her that they would return for her "when the time is right." Maggie thought this vision was a riot. The content may have been incongruous, but that didn't affect her positivity and equanimity. She remained just as secure in love and meaning at life's end as at its beginning.

Maggie's deceased parents as well as her beloved sister Beth came to her very early within the course of her illness—weeks, not days, before her passing. In the world of her pre-death dreams, her loved ones served as guides, giving her the direction and reassurance the larger world couldn't. They informed her, "It's not your time yet," and said, "We will come back for you." Strikingly, the fact that they were deceased seemed irrelevant to Maggie. What mattered was that their love and support still resonated with her. To Maggie, these feelings were undeniably real.

Unlike patients such as Patricia, Maggie did not speak of her end-of-life experiences objectively. She did not evaluate them critically. For her, these events were lived and cherished from within. Where her mind may have lagged, her heart did not—it led with fury. The vividness and potency with which she experienced her end-of-life dreams and visions became particularly visible during an interview that was captured on film.

As Maggie began to describe her dream of her deceased sister Beth's return, her lighthearted manner faded, and she was overcome with emotion. In her own words, "I was in bed when my sister came to me, the one who died." As she continued to describe the dream events, Maggie sounded distressed, and her breathing became laden with emotion. As with so many others who describe their inner-world experience, the line between the imagined world and her reality was blurred in the telling. In her dream, Maggie was pleading to her sister, "Stay with me, don't leave me." Beth replied, "I just can't; I can't stay with you." Even as she relayed these words, Maggie began to cry, struggling to find her voice. She recalled pleading with her sister again, "Beth, you're going to stay with me? I am alone, stay with me."

As Maggie reexperienced the scene, time and distance again became irrelevant. And just as her parents had provided gentle reassurance, her sister replied, "I can't. Not now. Soon we'll be together." The dream ended with Beth's soothing plea that her dying sister "just lie down." As Maggie repeated her sister's final request, her composure returned, and the tears stopped flowing. She was no longer sad.

What impressed me, then as much as now, is that Maggie's end-of-life experience not only challenges but inverts our common assumptions about dying. From our vantage point, most of us readily identify with the poet Dylan Thomas's exhortation not to "go gentle into that good night . . . Rage, rage against the dying of the light." The sentiment is as beautiful as it is lyrical, but it may not describe dying accurately. Whereas Thomas could only imagine death, Maggie was actually experiencing it. For her, dying had absolutely nothing to do with rage. She was not fighting "against the dying of the light"; her struggle was to get back to her childhood home in Buffalo.

For Maggie, dying was inseparable from where she grew up, lived, became ill, and would die, all within the same emotional net tightly woven by her loving family. She was never alone, no more in dying than in life. Her end-of-life experiences not only diminished her fear of death but also restored her sense of connectedness and belonging.

Mahatma Gandhi once described happiness as a state in which "what you think, what you say and what you do are in harmony." The statement could not more aptly describe the extraordinary woman Maggie was. While the outside world mostly saw a mismatch between who she was and who she should be, her inner life and its manifestation in her end-of-life dreams showed how attuned she was, both to herself and to others.

Unfortunately, many patients whose cognitive impairment is more severe arrive at the end of life without the kind of alignment of inner and outer selves that defined living for Maggie.

Instead, these patients are estranged from their core self. The loss of cognitive functioning often referred to as Alzheimer's dementia is an extreme example of that condition. The disease separates us in irredeemable ways from ourselves, or from what the neurologist Oliver Sacks referred to as the "inner state." Unlike other afflictions, Alzheimer's dementia creates a world where cognition unravels, yet emotions and senses remain intact.

People with dementia are typically excluded from formal research studies, which depend on the patient having intact cognition in order to provide informed consent. But, if we are to do justice to the entirety of the human experience at life's end, we need to include patients with dementia. And of course, disentangling the world of those suffering from dementia also entails considering the caregiver on whom they depend to navigate an unrecognizable world.

The descent into dementia typically leads to a disproportionate clinical focus on the patient's challenging behaviors and their management, to the detriment of the person's buried psychological states of being. The clinical world may also inadvertently be obscuring the subjective world of those with dementia by only considering the loss of measurable cognitive abilities. This happens because clinicians are often only drawn to observable behaviors and evidence of defectiveness. The clinical nomenclature of deficit becomes the currency through which we discuss patients, as we become overly reliant on assessing people's inability to repeat numbers or recall the names of past presidents. In so doing, we ignore the view from inside, the richness within the subjective states of dementia. We fail to consider the lived experiences of people with dementia because we let our awareness of their condition obscure their personhood.

Although it is true that the details and facts of much of their earlier lives may be lost, the defining emotional richness of having lived often persists in the inner world of those with brain disorders. It is not uncommon for an Alzheimer's patient to remember the name of their childhood dog and not recall the day of the week. That is because dementia impairs the ability to form new memories. The disease is unusually cruel for people like my friend Dr. John Tangeman, whose mother suffered a traumatic early life and was therefore cursed to relive a painful past rather than her more hopeful and forgiving present.

Gerd Vaagen was born in 1925 in Ålesund, Norway, to a sea captain and a housewife. She had an idyllic childhood, which included Alpine skiing on a magnificent mountain range in winter, and aquatic sports and sailing in the local fjords during the summer. Gerd was a freshman in high school when the Nazis invaded Norway on April 9, 1940. She saw her country become the most heavily fortified nation during the war, with a ratio of one German soldier for every eight Norwegians.

What followed was a five-year occupation by the Wehrmacht that led to German-imposed food shortages, the wide censorship of the press, and a blatantly improbable Nazi propaganda that tried, for instance, to rebrand the well-known "heil" salute as an ancient Norwegian tradition dating back to the Vikings.

Gerd witnessed horrors that would haunt her for the rest of her life. She saw her school principal summarily executed when he was caught with a radio transmitter. She lost numerous friends who had become involved in the resistance movement. Her family suffered from what bordered on famine. Her father even had a physician place a cast on her arm, which she wore for a year for a nonexistent deformity. He wanted to mark his daughter as defective, so she would not become part of the Lebensborn project of Nazi eugenics. This consisted of occupying Germans impregnating healthy and blond, blue-eyed women to "purify" the Aryan race.

After the war, Gerd's life was tragically marked by continued trauma and loss. She had just completed a master's degree in library science at Oxford when her high school sweetheart and husband died in a sailing accident. He was only in his twenties. In 1954, in an effort to leave the past behind, Gerd left her family and friends to travel to the United States. She eventually remarried and settled in Buffalo, where she had two sons, the younger of whom, Thomas, died of leukemia at age three. When Gerd was fifty-two, her second husband died unexpectedly, and the family of four became two.

My colleague John, Gerd's second son, remembers to this day his mother's lifelong grief as well as her anger and bitterness toward the war and those who waged it. Family gatherings used to begin with pleas to limit the reliving of Nazi atrocities. The trauma of the war consumed much of her identity and only worsened with the loss of her husband, John's father. Early on in the course of her dementia, Gerd became ever more obsessed with memories of the war, so much so that she believed Hitler himself was directly to blame for any frustration that occurred during the day, from a meal served cold to a lost TV remote.

Dementia is particularly challenging for close family members, who progressively lose the person they once held dear and no longer recognize. They watch powerlessly as their relative gradually becomes a shell of their former self. John could not help but feel a sense of abandonment in Gerd's very presence. He felt robbed of his relationship with her, so much so that he began grieving his mother's loss long before her death.

As the years passed and death drew near, an unusual transformation took place that gradually erased the bitterness and anger that had so dominated Gerd's life. Hitler's ill-doings were forgotten, and the terrors of the war gave way to an extraordinary sense of composure. Gerd also became uncharacteristically pleasant and demonstrably affectionate with those providing care. Instead of living within the confines of past anguish, she spent hours staring lovingly at the portrait of her deceased son Thomas. John would often find his mother blowing kisses to his late brother's picture, recalling the good years, and professing her undying love. Gerd was reclaiming her long-departed son.

As her dementia progressed, the burden of her life's memories was lifted and she seemed to be the person she was before her memories of trauma took over. Her transformation was so complete that she would become frightened at her own image in the mirror, which she referred to as the "crazy lady." John eventually had to cover the mirror with a cloth to spare her feelings. She was now so anchored to a distant past that she could no longer recognize her own eighty-five-year-old reflection, or maybe she was rejecting what she saw as a representation of her damaged soul.

Gerd died peacefully several weeks later. She may have lived with a distorted notion of reality but, in her last moments, she returned to the one memory that had brought her closer to a less damaged sense of self and released her from her anguish.

For patients suffering from Alzheimer's and other dementias, the line between end-of-life experiences in sleep versus wakefulness is even more blurred than the reality they can no longer share. And because people with dementia exist within an unshared world, their dream experiences ultimately remain their secret. Yet these patients also frequently undergo inner changes as part of the dying process. It may be that they are healing old wounds, exploring what's lost, or reclaiming a distant love. We may not be able to collect evidence to prove it—at any rate, not of the kind that would withstand scientific scrutiny—but I have seen the process unravel again and again. I have witnessed patients with severe cognitive loss paradoxically experience a vibrant and rejuvenating inner life in the process of dying.

Physicians such as Oliver Sacks have noted that those with dementia have an emotional intelligence that can be unlocked with the right key, such as music, for instance. This emphasis on the creative arts underscores the error commonly made in evaluating patients based on their capacity to reason rather than to feel. Their minds may be lost to us, but they still resonate within themselves. Nor can they be separated from their heart and its capacity for love.

Down syndrome too is one of the conditions that often lead to misconceptions about how or whether affected people process the larger meanings of death and dying. Assumptions are made about how they may or may not respond to a terminal diagnosis and what information should be shared. I don't presume to have answers to these questions, but I have witnessed in such patients a remarkable resilience, an ability to cultivate peace as well as find meaning within their illness.

End-of-life experiences in particular have the potential to

help the dying reach emotions that may not be accessible otherwise. This was the case for a patient named Sammy for whom I cared in the last few months of her life. Sammy had Down syndrome and was diagnosed with metastatic ovarian cancer at age thirty-six. She and I frequently talked about her illness and the need to treat her symptoms. The disease had caused her belly to protrude from ascites, the medical name for a large amount of fluid accumulation in the abdomen. I would try to address her condition, and she would immediately correct me: "It is because I am pregnant." Sammy had transcended the grim reality of her terminal diagnosis by reassigning the source of her physical discomfort. When I inquired about the severity of the nausea, stomach pain, and fatigue that accompanied her condition, she smiled and insisted, "I know. It is because I am pregnant." As her illness progressed, her discomfort increased and so did the size of her abdomen, which only reinforced her joy in the anticipation of motherhood. And when she slept, her dreams only confirmed her alternate reality.

I began to worry how others might respond to or redefine Sammy's interpretation of her illness. She lived in a residential home for people with disabilities who could only be described as her extended family. The home was not fancy, but it was clean, reliable, and safe. Over the previous few years, I had been at that particular residence several times to check on patients. I recognized many of the staff and soon realized that my concern for Sammy was misplaced. The people who do direct care typically develop remarkable clinical insight and judgment. The staff in Sammy's home excelled in their hybrid role of providing a familiar and reassuring presence while gently guiding residents through the motions of the day.

Sammy rarely received outside visitors, but she had made herself part of the "family" she had joined almost a decade earlier. Until recently, she had managed most of the daily activities on her own and enjoyed the organized outings to the mall as well as the life-skills-based training regularly provided the residents. As my visits multiplied, she would tell me at length about the cooking and money-management tips she had been given in one workshop or another. I probably had more use for them than she realized.

In the absence of blood relatives, Sammy had gone and set the stage for an imaginary one. Her disability had denied her motherhood but not a maternal instinct. She had held and carried dolls around all her life and the staff often soothed Sammy by providing her with replicas of a baby. The latest had a cuddly cloth body with chubby arms and legs made out of a skin-toned material. But at death's door, Sammy was no longer willing to settle for substitutes. Despite the medication, imaging, lab tests, and hospital visits, she had turned symptoms of her illness into evidence of the presence of a baby: "I am pregnant." End of story. And maybe more importantly, it was *her* story, and she was sticking to it.

Sammy had rewritten dying, or the losing of life, as the giving of life. It was what she had always wanted, the resolution to the unmet need she had carried for decades alongside her doll.

I remember discussing the details of her pain management a few days before her death, only to have her smile and repeat her mantra, "That is okay, Dr. Kerr. It is just the baby acting out." I smiled back, holding her gaze, grateful for the magical process through which our inner worlds prevail to address our deepest wishes. Sammy, like Maggie, was a true miracle to me.

Taking care of her also meant reconsidering the hypothesis with which I started this chapter—the notion that end-of-life experiences are universal irrespective of cognitive or neurodevelopmental status. I had reproduced the unconscious bias that we sometimes apply to people who are different. I was looking for sameness, an unhelpful and limiting comparison between "them" and "us." Sammy showed me the extent to which sameness is irrelevant. Her end-of-life experiences were as unique as she was, and the gap between her perception and others' did not amount to a lesser experience. In fact, Sammy's end-of-life experiences were arguably more potent because of the continuity they maintained with her long-held image and the fact that they were as real to her whether she was awake or asleep.

Where Sammy helped me sketch a more accurate picture of how the cognitively different experience dying, Andre, a man with autism, completed it. He provided yet another powerful reminder that conclusions and conjecture surrounding end of life can only be accurate if they draw on patient testimony.

As a high-functioning autistic man, Andre had worked as a bag boy at a local grocery store for most of his life. After his parents died, he had been cared for by his cousin Lisa's parents, and years later, when she became a mother of three, he was again integrated into her family. Even as an adult, Andre required a certain level of dependence on others, but his care, like Maggie's, had always translated into belonging, not burden. Andre enriched the three generations of family by giving as much love as he received.

His purity of heart and joyfulness grounded his strong and easy identification with children. Lisa's son Hazen was three years old when Andre moved in, and the two connected instantly. They became inseparable, the best of friends, playing Nerf guns around the house, communicating with walkie-talkies from different rooms, dressing up for Halloween, carving pumpkins, and hiding under piles of leaves in the yard. Andre loved family trips and Easter egg hunts. His family described him as "childlike" but also respected his strong sense of independence. He could put together breakfast, make his own lunch for work, and buy things in the store with little to no help. Andre would live with Lisa's family for the next thirteen years, until his death at seventy-five.

When Lisa reminisces about the place Andre occupied in their hearts and lives, it is with overwhelming and grateful emotion. She will explain that, with Andre, her children learned invaluable lessons in empathy. Having him in their young lives meant intuitively knowing when to step in and assist, and he in turn provided them with unconditional love and laughter.

In May 2017, Andre, then seventy-four, was diagnosed with congestive heart failure and bladder cancer. Hospice care was recommended. The doctors estimated that it would be his heart, not the cancer, that would eventually cause his death. None of this was shared with Andre, who went on to live happily and unencumbered until his stroke on December 1, 2017.

Lisa and her husband, Merle, focused on helping Andre live each day to the fullest. At this time, he was using a walker and had a catheter bag 24/7, but he always smiled and met each day with a sense of wonder. He lived without a full awareness of his terminal status. This is why it was so moving to Lisa when a month before he died, he started seeing what she later identified as deceased relatives. It was always during the daytime hours, and she could tell when it occurred because he would stare at the window with big, open eyes. In these moments, Merle noted that Andre seemed to "perk up" with an "excitable curiosity," which he immediately wanted to share.

The first time, he saw a man with a hat. Andre didn't recognize him, but he was a friendly presence who waved at him. The next time, it was a man and a woman, and he thought the woman looked vaguely familiar, maybe like a grandmother. The "visits" happened almost daily. He once saw another man taking pictures, which also happened to be Andre's favorite hobby.

On another occasion, it was Lisa's deceased mom he saw in the room and pointed to while talking to his second cousin. She was sitting on his suitcase, Andre exclaimed with a laugh. Like two-thirds of our patients, his end-of-life experiences included themes of preparing to go, either through travel or packing.

To Lisa, Andre's most moving vision was the one he had of her nephew Lucas as a boy. It was fitting that Andre's end-of-life experiences would reflect his fondness for children. Lucas had died at almost six years old from an aggressive form of leukemia. He was the same age as Lisa's daughter Gabrielle, with whom he had grown up. The two kids were inseparable, and their favorite thing in the world was to catch butterflies. Andre's vision included a child chasing butterflies, but it was much more than a snapshot of a past attachment. It also carried a message, which he matter-of-factly relayed to Lisa: "He told me that he had died." This was how Andre's end-of-life experiences most effectively familiarized him with the imminence of death, making it as conceivable and harmless as chasing butterflies.

Andre lived these pre-death experiences as if they were

natural extensions of his everyday life. He never paused to wonder whether or why he was dreaming. He didn't ask who these people were. He was not worried about what it could possibly mean. He just knew at an intuitive level that these were positive experiences that made him feel good. He felt secure, surrounded, loved. And he giggled.

For Lisa and Merle, being able to share Andre's end-of-life experiences, sometimes through the photo albums and pictures in which he recognized a face, was an unforgettable time of togetherness. Their daughter Gabrielle was similarly moved; the remembrances allowed her to revisit the happy memories of her preteen years without having to relive the tragic loss of her beloved cousin Lucas. The whole family found comfort in knowing that Andre was blessed with end-of-life experiences that helped him transition with what he cherished most, a sense of belonging. Andre's last end-of-life experiences were not only comforting to him but, in Lisa's words, also "welcoming." Lisa commented that while "so many are on drugs for pain at the end, Andre was not." In fact, he was "fully awake" up until two days before his death.

Whereas most of us exist with clearly defined boundaries between what we perceive as reality and what our inner life and unconscious tell us, Andre moved seamlessly between the two. For him, as for Sammy, pre-death dreams were less about a new, emerging consciousness that had to be reconciled with his surroundings than an extension of the emotional clarity that had always defined his life and relationships. Just as Sammy's mothering instinct never once wavered, Andre's end-of-life experiences represented a continued reflection of who he was. His persona never varied with circumstance, and his disposition remained as beautiful as it was true. Unlike those of us whose end-of-life experiences may be remembered with psychological and emotional processes through which we need to find our way, Andre's experience was a straightforward journey through grace.

I do not have any special access to the perspectives of those we identify as disabled, any more than I do to the end-of-life experiences of any other patient who is unable to share them. But it would be false to say this process leaves no trace. At its best, palliative care is about being wholly present as we are brought to witness the unique essence of each person's light, no matter how faint it is or how different they are. In fact, what occurs in the recesses of the heart and mind at life's end may never be wholly accessible to others, no matter how abled or disabled the person is considered to be.

In the prophetic words of novelist Franz Kafka, "It is entirely conceivable that life's splendor lies in wait about each one of us in all its fullness, but veiled from our point of view, deep down, far off. . . . This is the essence of magic, which does not create but summons."

# to those left behind

You didn't die
you just changed shape
became invisible
to the naked eye
became this grief
its sharpness
more real
than your presence was
before you were separate to me
entire to yourself
now you are
a part of me
you are inside my self

—DÓNALL DEMPSEY

*When Breath Becomes Air*, Paul Kalanithi's haunting memoir about battling lung cancer, concludes with the moving tribute his wife wrote following his premature death. Lucy Kalanithi describes how, two days before her husband's passing, "My heart swelled even as I steeled myself, anticipating his suffering, worrying that he had only weeks left. . . . I didn't know that Paul would die within days." And as she takes stock of the severity of his condition, she is overcome with grief: "I already missed him."

Lucy's experience of mourning belies our understanding of bereavement as what happens *after* the loss of a loved one. For her, grief entailed no clear onset for the beginning or end of her feelings of loss, no identifiable moment separating dying from death, presence from absence, the before from the after.

The human grief experience is multidimensional, flexible, and personal. Bereaved family members and caregivers learn to adjust to a world bereft of their loved one in myriad ways that are not neatly aligned with our usual temporal markers. What remains a constant, however, is the higher level of acceptance achieved by the bereaved when their dying loved one is at peace. We derive comfort and reassurance from the knowledge that our family members felt at ease in their last moments. This is what happens, for instance, when those left behind witness the life-affirming effects of end-of-life experiences in their dying relatives. The more positive the bereaved perceive end-of-life experiences to be for dying patients, the more it helps them work through the pain of their own grief. In the words of the elderly sister of one of our patients, "When he told me that he saw his favorite sister [deceased] hold out her hands to him, it made me feel comforted because I knew it comforted him. He loved her very much and she adored him." Caregivers repeatedly may even use words that denote contentment rather than mourning: "He did find comfort talking to and seeing people who passed before him. He was not afraid or scared—he had told me," or, "I still remember [these dreams] and enjoy the memories."

Sometimes, pre-death dreams help survivors by uncovering aspects of the patient's past that were long hidden from view. It was thanks to his end-of-life experiences that John Stinson's family got to meet the man they had never known, the twenty-year-old soldier who would one day become their father. By the time he was eighty-seven, John had fought his whole life to suppress his experience of war. He had never told his family about the horrors he had witnessed during his rescue mission on the shores of Normandy and suffered silently until his final days, when distant memories fought to surface.

"I learned more about my dad in the last two weeks than I did during his lifetime," John's son explained while reminiscing about his father's end-of-life reckoning. His sister corroborated the sentiment: "My brother, as well as the rest of us, knew very little about my father's war experience. He rarely spoke of that time in his life. Some of what we learned in those last few weeks of his life we had never heard before. He just never really talked to us about it!" They may have been in the dark about the details of the past their father was revisiting, but not about the positive outcome of what transpired on his deathbed. Several years after their dad's passing, the account of his peaceful transition still brought tears of gratitude to their eyes.

For twenty-eight-year-old Sierra's family, grieving began in a daze, in the little to no time they all had to adjust to the knowledge of her imminent death. Sierra's abdominal discomfort was first misdiagnosed as appendicitis. By the time further tests were ordered, they revealed a diagnosis of widely metastasized colon cancer. Her mother, Tammy, still remembers the incomprehensible calm with which Sierra received the terrible news. Tammy's agony, as a parent, was compounded by the perception that Sierra seemed to be in denial about the severity of her own condition.

At the cancer hospital where she was undergoing chemotherapy, Sierra began planning her wedding, the one she had always dreamt of, to the father of her four-year-old son. The oncologist finally took her mother aside to suggest they not wait the two months Sierra thought she needed to make the arrangements. Unable to comfort her daughter, a heartbroken Tammy found herself begging Sierra's fiancé to move up the date of a wedding he had suggested but did not truly want. It was not to be. Less than two months elapsed between the trauma of the diagnosis and Sierra's admission to Hospice Buffalo, where she was transferred from the cancer hospital with just days to live. There had literally been no time to process the implications of transitioning from hospitalized treatment to palliative care, let alone from wedding to dying. "I am going to beat this," she still insistently told the hospice doctors and nurses.

Sierra's pain was unrelenting and her condition rapidly deteriorated. Symptom management was prioritized, but it was also urgent to help her and her family understand that her time was limited so that they could reach some level of acceptance and find the words to say their final good-byes. Although we knew that end-of-life dreams and visions help patients come to terms with death, in Sierra's case we just assumed that her denial meant the absence of such experiences.

Sierra's medical team, including palliative care physician

Dr. Megan Farrell, the chaplain, the nurses, and the social worker, decided to stage an intervention of sorts. They first met with Tammy and Sierra's siblings, who ranged in age from eight to twenty-six years. Sierra's stepfather was also present. The family's shock at hearing a doctor verbalize the reality of Sierra's approaching death was palpable, but it was also softened by the loving testimonies about her life that soon filled the room. Toward the end of the meeting, Dr. Farrell asked one of the older siblings how Sierra made sense of what was happening to her. The answer came in a flurry of tears: "She really thinks she is going to beat this. She does not believe she's dying."

The first step on the path to peace in grieving as well as in dying is acceptance. Sierra was struggling to reconcile the different realities that were clashing around her. She needed clarity about her condition so that she could acknowledge the inevitable. This was something that the science of medicine alone could not bring forth. It was also a process of understanding that, unbeknownst to her caretakers, Sierra's end-of-life experiences had already initiated. In bypassing language altogether, they were preparing her for the reality that her loved ones were so hesitant to put into words.

The next day, Sierra's parents and caretakers all gathered around her bed for the dreaded talk. Dr. Farrell spoke first. She expressed her personal regret that "despite my best efforts and those of your other doctors, we haven't been able to fix the underlying problem and rid you of the disease that has taken such a toll on you." Sierra admitted that she felt weaker, but she remained steadfast in her defiance in the face of impending death: "I'm going to beat this," she whispered feebly. Tammy was choking back sobs.

Dr. Farrell moved closer to her patient. She acknowledged how hard Sierra had been struggling for her mom, her son, and her family. She affirmed the overwhelming love and care that permeated the room. Then she gently asked, "Sierra, do you think about the future?" The answer came, wordless, in the form of big tears that began coursing down Sierra's cheeks. Tammy held back a mother's impulse to wipe them away.

Dr. Farrell then asked Sierra if she'd had any dreams. "Yes, strange dreams," her young patient answered, "and they don't always make sense. Sometimes I don't remember them very well." The physician continued, "Sierra, is there anyone you have been dreaming about or someone in particular who comes to you in your dreams?"

A long pause ensued. With eyes half open, Sierra looked over her doctor's shoulder, smiled, and whispered, "Hi, Grandpa!"

Tammy began weeping. This was not the first time that Sierra had been dreaming of her grandpa Howard, a decorated army veteran and a devoted family man who had been particularly close to his beloved granddaughter. Grandpa Howard had appeared in Sierra's dreams at the cancer center, but now, in the stillness of her hospice room, surrounded by loved ones in this moment of impossible truth, Sierra's vision of him represented so much more than just a recurring dream. It was a manifestation of a state of being that brought clarity and made words such as *terminal illness* and *dying* irrelevant. It was what made everyone understand a language we knew but did not speak, one in which feeling and knowing merged into one. It was also what would help Tammy release the burden of her broken heart.

Everyone was speechless. Tammy broke the silence: "Sierra, what is Grandpa saying?"

"He says he is proud of the young woman and mother I have become," Sierra answered slowly but distinctly. She was drifting in and out of consciousness. "He does not want me to suffer." Those were the whispered words that let Tammy know that she needed to give her daughter permission to let go.

"When Grandpa comes for you, you go with him, baby girl. Don't worry about us," she heard herself tell Sierra, with a firm selflessness and strength she did not know she could muster.

This powerful scene was one no one present would ever forget. They had entered the room with years of experience in multiple disciplines, from spiritual to medical care, hoping to help Sierra come to terms with her impending death. Instead, their patient had asserted her own understanding of mortality. They had come to stage an intervention but had been subjected to one themselves, a reminder that the best lessons are often witnessed, not taught.

Sierra died four days later, surrounded by her loving family and friends. She took her last breath in her mother's arms, after Tammy climbed into her child's deathbed to hold her just a little while longer. Sometimes it takes holding on tight to let go. To the grieving mother, it was both "profound and surreal" to know that she had somehow excruciatingly come full circle with her youngest child: "I was there when she took her first breath, and I was there when she took her last. Not many parents can say that."

Although it stands to reason that end-of-life experiences, in helping the patient find comfort, also benefit the loved ones, the impact of dreams on bereavement has largely gone unexamined. Not only has limited research been conducted from the perspective of the patient, but until recently only one study, in

Japan, has examined the effect of end-of-life dreams on the grieving family. This gap may be one of the most troubling legacies of a scientific approach that dismisses any subjective dimension as suspect, whether it is that of the patient or the caregiver.

In a recent study on bereavement conducted at Hospice Buffalo, more than half the participants (54 percent) whose loved ones had experienced pre-death dreams and visions confirmed that this knowledge influenced their overall grief journey. One family caregiver shared, "We both believed from the beginning that he would be in a better place; that our love endured throughout. His vision of his 'grave' pleased him—gave him comfort. He did envision the transition place—he was at peace. I don't feel he is gone. Changed, yes, but always present—there somehow." Others expressed similar positive outcomes of sharing dreams and finding comfort in them. "My mom's vision was happy and peaceful. She was glad, welcomed who she was interacting with. I knew she was leaving us and happy to leave. Her visions were very comforting to her, and us." Their loved ones' end-of-life experiences helped the bereaved accept the reality of the loss because "her acceptance . . . made everything easier." In fact, the more comforting caregivers believe pre-death dreams and visions to be for their dying relatives, the more soothed they feel about their own loss, both on a short- and long-term basis. Solace for the dying consistently translates into comfort and peace for the caregivers. Bereavement may not be a straightforward journey as it unravels alongside the dying process, but it need not be wholly deprived of light. It is important to recognize and honor how the mourning process the patient's family goes through is aided by the dying loved one's end-of-life experiences.

It may have been a loving grandparent that Sierra summoned to help the family transition to acceptance, but the final guides conjured by pre-death dreams and visions are not always older or even wiser relatives. Sometimes, death's attendant is as young as a baby. The currency of life is not age or experience, but the love given and the love received.

When his wife was admitted to hospice, eighty-one-year-old Robert told me on several occasions that he wished he were first to go. He could not cope with losing Barbara, his partner of sixty years, and was overcome with conflicted feelings of guilt, loss, despair, and also faith. He put up a brave front in Barbara's presence but came undone as soon as he left her bedside. One day, however, she had a vision of the baby boy they had lost decades before. Like Mary, whose similar gesture had once startled me, Barbara was reaching for her son and smiling blissfully during a short span of lucid dreaming. It was a moment of pure wholeness and grace, one that Robert had no trouble recognizing as such. The scene brought about a genuine turning point in his grieving process. Observing his wife's dreaming provided Robert with a life-affirming feeling in the midst of his irredeemable loss. In fact, both husband and wife were transformed in its aftermath, becoming more peaceful and able to enjoy the remainder of the time they had together. It was clear that Barbara was experiencing her imminent passing as a time of love regained, and seeing her comforted brought Robert peace.

The bereaved are often most troubled by a simple question: is their dying loved one going to be okay? Another husband of a patient, Paul, also took great comfort in the realization that his dying wife Joyce's dreams helped resurrect the love that had sustained her the most in childhood: her father's. He realized then that she was finally at peace and he was able to let her go.

Years later when Paul, in turn, became a patient in our home hospice care program, that knowledge was still reverberating within him, helping him approach his own death with equanimity. He was at ease even before he began having visions of his deceased wife. His most recurrent dream was that of Joyce, in her favorite blue dress, waving at him. He told me how she'd given him "the little beauty pageant wave" to let him know that she was fine and that he'd be fine too.

Paul enjoyed sharing his experiences, and his daughter, Diane, a nurse, was heartened to hear him talk about his end-of-life dreams. She shared that he would "get a lot out of it. He chose to remember the positive dreams that he had, so we all enjoyed always hearing about Dad's dreams. I could always take my cues from Dad. If Dad was comforted by those dreams, that is what I was looking for. My father's last few days on earth were the last gift that he gave us as a father. Because of circumstances from the past, as soon as Dad had a stroke, four and a half days before he died, everybody raced to get there. Two of my brothers were not able to be with us when my mother died and it was important to all [seven] of us to be here now. And we spent four days in our childhood home, providing care for my father, people in and out, cooking for each other, taking care of Dad, visiting with Dad, priests came and went, family members came and went, friends and neighbors came and went, and we were given the greatest gift to know that we were all going to be together, that Dad might not be there but he brought us all together one more time and we took that with us; that was a tremendous gift he gave us. He couldn't speak, but he could smile, and there was light in his eyes. He was there with us until the last couple of hours before he died."

The greatest fear a dying patient's family faces often mirrors that of the patient. They too want to know if their loved one is at peace. Where do their minds and hearts drift when they can't speak and have closed their eyes? Paul's pre-death experiences helped answer these questions and more. He was returned to love.

Pre-death dreams and visions assist loved ones in their journey toward acceptance—the key to processing loss. They help fill the void that may be created by emptiness, doubt, or fear. When the dying patient becomes absorbed in and then comforted by their end-of-life experiences, it changes the context of dying from loneliness to a life-affirming connection. And this is as significant for the bereaved as it is for the dying.

Bereaved family members sometimes benefit from the soothing effects of their dying relative's end-of-life experiences years down the line. At the threshold of death, Dwayne, the lifelong addict who had become estranged from his daughter Brittany, underwent a transformation that carried over into his daughter's life. It was their deathbed reunion, and the forgiveness that flowed from their love, that helped Brittany forge a commitment to turn her life around.

This reconciliation emanated from the person who paid the highest price for Dwayne's lifetime of addiction: his adoring daughter. For Brittany, her father's disease had meant growing up with an absentee dad and landing in the foster care system, where she was subjected to years of abuse. It had meant running away at age fourteen and spending three years in juvenile detention. It had meant relying on the only source of comfort that her father had known and modeled: drugs and dependence. Dwayne did not believe himself deserving of forgiveness, nor did Brittany necessarily think herself capable of it. But when father and daughter reunited, he'd had "dreams of reckoning" that had changed his whole perspective. He desperately wanted to make amends and was sincere in his yearning for reconciliation. And for Brittany, that made all the difference.

The man who emerged from experiencing the most harrowing end-of-life dreams was the dad Brittany chose to remember, not the father who had abandoned his children: "All my sisters, we all have different fathers except for the last two; every single one of us called him Dad. He was a father to all of us. Despite all his mishaps, I don't have no regrets of him being my father. If you asked me, it never happened. It never happened because he wasn't that type of person. I don't have a bad word to say about him." The only side of Dwayne that now mattered to her was the dad who told her how to love herself and said, "You are my baby." She continued: "Don't follow the streets; there is nothing in the streets. Always be a woman who respects yourself, always love your family, never put nothing before something that you love and you can benefit from."

Dwayne himself credited his apocalyptic dreams for his end-of-life transformation and its ensuing impact on his daughter. So did Brittany: "I think by him having those dreams it was a sign. [Without the dreams] he would have been all stressed out about his health instead of worrying about the people who he had hurt. Maybe he needed to have those dreams."

Dwayne's end-of-life experiences truly had a ripple effect whose impact lasted long after his death. And in honor of the father who had changed the course of his life, albeit at the eleventh hour, Brittany set out to do the same.

We reconnected with Brittany two years after her father's passing, in the context of the interview for the documentary on end-of-life dreams. Now twenty-seven, she still had the same breezy and charismatic personality that spelled joy. She had a steady job, loyal friends, and a sense of purpose. A true extrovert, she immediately took charge of the interview and was the one to set everyone at ease when memories of her late father brought tears to her eyes. Brittany was grateful that we were "taking the time out to see what type of person my dad really was when you didn't know him from a can of paint." No one except her grandmother and her sibling mentioned him anymore, so to see us so engaged with his memory moved her to tears. "Most people didn't care about him," she added. "They only talked about what they saw and heard. I don't care what nobody say about my dad, can't nobody tell me anything about my dad. I don't care what he did." But she did care. She cared that the criminal she had once referred to as her father had finally changed into the man who deserved to be called Dad.

Brittany had needed no tangible proof to know that her father, weak and dying as he was, had changed in profound and irrevocable ways, and this in turn sustained her in the knowledge that his passing would be serene. She was so fiercely proud of him that she scoffed at our offer to change his name for the book and documentary. "We are not fake," she responded with her head held high. I explained that there might be very legitimate reasons to protect her identity that did not involve shame or hypocrisy, but she insisted. "It's Dwayne Earl Johnson. Dwayne. Earl. Johnson," she repeated with a voice that enveloped us with its warmth and dignity. I expected her to point to her tattoo of "Dad," with his dates of birth and death, and "RIP" displayed on her forearm, but she never did. She did not need to exhibit her love; it was just part of her.

End-of-life dreams and visions may be experiences limited to the inner life, without visible material effects, but their impact is no less potent for being unseen. There are times when they even transcend generations to meet unaddressed spiritual and emotional needs, those that tie a parent to a child and that restore once-forsaken bonds. And then there are times when such experiences do not influence the reality of the bereaved so much as replace it. This often happens with elderly couples who, following a lifetime of togetherness, cannot shift to living without their other half. And so they don't. Instead, they maintain their unbreakable bond through end-of-life experiences. Attention switches to the inner world, where they go on coexisting with their deceased partners and can feel whole again. That is when bereavement does not involve a before and an after, only a different and in some ways deeper bond.

Lisa, Sonny and Joan's daughter and caregiver, did not realize the tremendous impact of her mother's end-of-life experiences until both of her parents had passed.

After Sonny's death, Joan kept her husband alive through pre-death visions that occurred in her dreams as well as when she was awake. As a result, it was only when she died that her daughter finally took stock of her double loss. Joan's end-of-life experiences had kept Sonny present not only as a husband but also as a father for his grieving daughter. And when the time came for Joan and Sonny to be reunited, the knowledge that their remarkable love story had survived death helped Lisa come to terms with her grief and sorrow. Her bereavement was aided by the recognition that her parents' bond had remained unbroken, thanks in large part to her mother's end-of-life experiences.

Feelings of grief are like feelings of love: they know no boundaries of time or space and spill over into areas of our lives we may not even be aware of; they are not only about the loss of a loved one but also about the self, either in the presence of the loved one or after. And even though bereavement follows no predictable or straightforward path, it is not necessarily deprived of light. It is important to honor the mourning process the patient's family goes through by recognizing how it is aided by the dying loved one's end-of-life experiences.

The power of dreams and visions in facilitating grieving is especially resonant when it comes to the bereaved parents of a young child. Both Kristin and Michele, Jess's and Ginny's moms, were distressed at the thought that death would be the only journey upon which their children would embark alone. There was nothing these mothers hadn't done for their daughters, these warrior moms, but now they were confronting the unbearable reality that there was nothing they could do.

No words can adequately describe the relief on the face of a parent who watches a dying child go from fear of the unknown to acceptance. For Michelle, it was Ginny's last dream that made her realize that even though the end was near, it would be a peaceful one. Indeed, following her pre-death dream about God, Ginny stopped calling out to Michele every fifteen minutes and started sleeping soundly. It was also in the wake of that dream that Michele felt inexplicably calm and settled, so much so that she finally found the strength to inquire about funeral arrangements. True to her warrior spirit, she wanted to attend to all remaining details so that her daughter's legacy could be properly honored.

Many bereaved family members make sense of their dying relative's end-of-life dreams and visions by drawing on a belief in God, angels, the afterlife, and heaven. That is what the rather agnostic Michele did after her daughter's last conversation with God. She questioned her own belief system, or lack thereof, while adopting the same language with which her daughter had made sense of her dying experience: "Who knows?" she said, smiling and throwing up her hands in surrender. "Maybe there is a castle. I no longer know what to believe." She, like many, turned to religion to explain Ginny's end-of-life experience even in light of her own lack of clear religious beliefs. Others turn to the supernatural simply in search of an "otherworldly" explanation. How each family chooses to understand the meaning of their loved ones' end-of-life dreams and visions matters little. What is remarkable is how, independent of our interpretive framework, the witnessing of these experiences helps the bereaved work through their pain of loss and accept the reality of separation.

Across dying and grieving, there remains a constant: the desire for connectivity. The therapeutic quality of end-of-life experiences extends to the bereaved in ways that can never be fully accounted for. For caregivers as much as for the dying, the possibility of being reunited allows them to adjust to life without their loved ones while maintaining a continuing bond. Whether its impact can be measured or not has no bearing on how undeniably powerful it is.

Kristin and Michele each responded to her child's death with the same remarkable disregard for the way it caused a form of separation. To this day, they each talk about and to their daughters on a daily basis. They each continue decorating their homes for the holidays for their little girls' sakes. They do it because "Ginny expects it" and "Jess would be upset with me if I ever skipped a year."

Three years after her daughter's passing, Kristin still smiles when pointing to the ornament her daughter had loosely affixed to the cat's collar on what turned out to be their last Christmas Eve together. The innocuous memento symbolizes a continued connection with her late daughter that cannot be severed by death and that grounds her and gives her the ability to come to terms with her inconceivable loss. As with Michele, Kristin finds the comfort she needs in her daughter's last end-of-life experience. In particular, Jess's vision of their deceased friend Mary, whom she identified as "an angel," is what provides Kristin with the reassurance that her little girl's transition mitigated its physical and emotional toll.

Like Kristen, Michele is still working through the pain of grief. She too was awed and comforted by her daughter's rich inner world and by the extraordinarily soothing quality of her end-of-life experiences. "She is always teaching me something," Michele said two days before Ginny's passing. She too continues to be moved by pictures, mementos, the toy animals that recall her daughter's presence. A rainbow appears and makes her smile. She sees heart shapes in clouds, rocks, even drops of water. The sight of a skunk conjures up the smell of Ginny's medication and makes her melancholy. A waitress's name is called out—"Ginny!"—and it startles her.

Michele often takes refuge in Ginny's room, which she has left untouched. The family cars are adorned with bumper stickers with Ginny's full name, Virginia Rose, and the dates of her birth and death. The mother takes her grief along with her wherever she goes, mostly because she has not had to repress or displace it. She does not cover up its challenges. Bereavement has become a steady and gentle companion, an extension of the therapeutic nature of Ginny's end-of-life experiences. Knowing that her daughter was soothed and peaceful at the end has made it possible for Michele to confront the unthinkable, and, with time, it has also helped turn shock into sadness, and trauma into grief.

In the midst of immense tragedy, Michele has found solace and meaning in small things, in scattered memories, and in the unbreakable bond she shared with her daughter. Hers is a love that keeps hoping and that transcends the waves of despair assailing her at irregular intervals. It is the same love that permeated her daughter's end-of-life experiences and whose cascading influence will sustain a heartbroken mother until the day she too finds her way to Ginny's castle.

Like most significant emotions, grief is not something we just get over; it is not something we can just go through in neat stages, and there is no prescribed order in which to handle it. It is something we move through, live and cope with, at times in stages, at other times in sudden bursts of emotion, protracted ebbs and flows, in despair but also in peace.

Ours are shared lives and histories, so it is not surprising that pre-death experiences embody this common reality. End of life makes visible the kind of light that signifies introspection and reflection and that goes on shining in darkness, even after grief has turned from a single event into a lifelong journey. It is a light that radiates far and wide and is felt when all language fails us.

—✳—

# beyond dream interpretation

*Life is not a problem to be solved, but a mystery to be lived.*

—THOMAS MERTON

Geraldine was a seventy-three-year-old retired prison guard with end-stage lung disease. When I first met her, she self-identified as an "ex–motorcycle chick." Geraldine showed little interest in uncovering the underlying meaning of her pre-death dreams, even when prompted to do so by well-meaning visitors like me. She did not pause to wonder about the coulds or should-have-beens of her existence. Instead, she described her pre-death dreams and visions with the amused detachment of a disinterested observer. Once she began telling me about her past, I understood why. She had lived through so much that nothing fazed her anymore.

Geraldine revealed harrowing details about childhood sexual abuse, years of neglect, abandonment, and multiple failed marriages marred by domestic violence and abandoned children, some abused, others estranged. Events that would make anyone's blood curdle made Geraldine chuckle. She had turned the traumas of her life into entertainment vignettes, stories to share and laugh about rather than process and overcome.

Trauma had left its mark, but Geraldine had fought back by turning it into the expected, the comical, even the banal. Maybe enacting the banality of trauma was the only way she knew how to distance herself from the hurt, or maybe it was due to her inability to process. Either way, Geraldine was a survivor, if nothing else. There were questions she could not afford to ask and answers she did not want to hear. After a life of emotional wounds left unattended and of meanings better left unexplored, she needed to feel love more than she needed to connect the dots.

Geraldine's long life had one identified love—unconditional, kind, and remembered—her mother. So her pre-death dreams turned to the only unsullied source of affection she had ever known, the "only one who cared" and who "is going to be there when I croak."

In their book *Dreaming Beyond Death: A Guide to Pre-Death Dreams and Visions*, Kelly Bulkeley and the Reverend Patricia Bulkley, who specialize in dream interpretation, also suggest that it is not always imperative for patients to interpret their pre-death dreams; sometimes it is best to sit with them, leaving them to do their work. This was certainly true for Geraldine. As caretakers of the dying, we know that sometimes the best help we can offer our patients is not to interfere at all but to merely be present. We know that to validate their dreams is not necessarily to interpret them. At life's end, Geraldine needed no intervention or explanation, no sense-making about the traumas she had experienced; she needed to register the one love she could relive in an authentic, unaffected manner. She felt supported, relieved, even joyful, when dreaming of her mother, and that is all that mattered.

When end-of-life experiences are discussed in the literature, it is typically through the lens of dream analysis, whether it is psychoanalysis (Freud) or analytical psychology (Carl Jung). As such, they are rarely distinguished from everyday dreams and get interpreted as projections of latent anxieties and desires or as coping mechanisms. They are seen as an enigma surrounding the patient's inner life, the key to which resides in dream interpretation; these approaches cast them as the beginning of a question in need of an answer.

By contrast, patients' end-of-life experiences provide answers to questions that no longer need asking. They represent a culminating point rather than a doorway. They are often blueprints for a peaceful, visionary, and certainly revisionist restaging of one's life whose impending end is only incidental to a pervasive sense of love. These experiences are not about thinking so much as about remembering, feeling, sensing, breathing, and smiling. They are about communication and connectivity, and they unravel in a realm that is best called transcendental. Indeed, in keeping with the meaning of *transcendence* as "going beyond," they take place on a plane that is radically different from anything that defines our ordinary, day-to-day, and ultimately finite experiences of living and dreaming. And although we talk about them as *dreams*, since that is the closest reference point we have to describe what happens at death's door, the longer I work with the dying, the less comfortable I am categorizing them as such. The phrase *end-of-life experiences* is truly a more accurate representation of a process that should not be confused with dreams experienced in health—or their interpretation, for that matter.

The fact is, I rarely meet patients in need of an interpretative approach to their pre-death dreams. End of life is no time for therapeutic interventions or quests for translation. The journey is over; we are behind the curtain. And it is worth asking whether the analysis of dreams is serving the needs of the clinician as opposed to the patient.

Sixty-seven years of introspection for a war veteran such as John Stinson did not accomplish what his end-of-life dream did in one night. Any critical distance between dreamer and the dream experience vanishes at death's door. Instead, what patients tell us loud and clear is that their end-of-life experiences differ from any dream they have ever had. They are more sensorial. They are deeply felt and lived. They feel "more real than real." When Geraldine described the sight of her mother's arms reaching out from above her bed, it was as a lived rather than imagined experience.

Even when patients do seek an explanation, the interpretation of their end-of-life experiences is hardly the point. The focus remains on how they feel, what they see, and how they are magically transported to a place of unparalleled love and support. Content matters less than the relations that are resurrected and the unique needs that are addressed. This may be the single most important distinction between regular dreams and pre-death dreams, and it points to the limitations of a psychoanalytic model when it comes to understanding the impact of end-of-life experiences.

It is because pre-death dreams are atypical that they are less amenable to the kind of interpretation applied to regular dreams. There is less symbolism, less abstraction, fewer behind-the-scene or underlying meanings. Very little is said between the dreamer and the people in the dream, while much is felt and inherently understood. Words appear less relevant and language of any kind is often unnecessary, as the larger meaning is intuited. In her dreams, it was not the two words Patricia uttered as a nine-year-old that carried the depth of meaning she shared with her dying mother in the impersonal hospital setting where she last saw her; and, as Jessica reminded me, that her dog Shadow could not talk—"Duh, Dr. Kerr!"—or even care to bark did not stop him from fulfilling his role as a trusted guide.

This is not to say that there is only ever one path to solace. Instead of protecting herself from answers, Rosemary worked hard to unearth them. Where Geraldine tried to evade meaning-making, Rosemary yearned for it. To her, pre-death dreams were something to take apart, analyze, explain, and understand. She went to bed intrigued, anxious for the night to unfold and reveal further truths about her end of life.

Rosemary was a seventy-year-old Buffalonian who had married her high school sweetheart and had lived and taught in the same community her whole life. When we approached her with our project study, she was thrilled to be able to represent the wisdom inherent in dying. She did so by relying on the craft she had honed throughout her professional life: writing. With death approaching, Rosemary set out to analyze her end-of-life experiences, diligently filling journal after journal with an account of her dreams and musings. True to her lifelong commitment to knowledge, she remained inquisitive till the very end. It was clear from her writings that she had wondered about the deeper meanings underlying her dreams and she wanted to interpret them for us. For instance, when she dreamt of standing outside a crowd of people, she teared up, explaining, "I am not sure what that means, exactly. I think it just means that I am leaving this world and all these other people are still going to be there." When she saw herself inside a funeral home, alone, she paused and said, "I don't know why I was there and who was there I would be visiting." She movingly described entering the funeral parlor filled with huge, beautiful flowers whose "gorgeous, gorgeous" colors she associated with the splendid and colorful silk scarves her daughter Beth made and dyed herself.

Rosemary's dreams felt so real to her that they brought her "much joy and happiness and part of that was that it was all about my daughter." They helped her not be afraid, she said. In creating meaning and reinforcing her values, they also helped her work out the transition from terror to acceptance, and from acceptance to love and comfort. After she died, we were touched to discover that she had bequeathed her journals to a member of our research team.

Rosemary and Geraldine both died as they had lived, which is also why they experienced and interpreted their pre-death dreams and visions in diametrically opposed ways. We often speak of death as the great equalizer but mistake equality with sameness, when it is because of our differences that equality matters. Even the categorization of people as *patients* assumes a likeness, when in fact the only commonality in being a patient is illness itself. Dying is more than the end point of disease; it is the closure of a life of which no two are the same. Where Rosemary worked hard to reconnect with her core self, Geraldine wanted to escape it. The former's engagement with end-of-life experiences was analytical, while the latter's was more intuitive. Yet both women were reacquainted with what was lost. They underwent a similar spiritual transformation whose outcome remained constant. Whether it was mother sees daughter or daughter sees mother, for both of them the theme was love. And each knew what to hold on to in order to put death into perspective or, in Rosemary's words, "to get on" with their lives.

End-of-life dreams and visions provide a path to peace no matter how or even whether they are interpreted. What matters is that they are lived, not examined. They embody the resilience with which the human spirit enters the dying process and makes it its own, independently of the way that transpires. Rosemary and Geraldine were two mothers with their share of life struggles, but, as different as they were, each displayed remarkable levelheadedness and strength in the face of adversity. And each shared a life story that went beyond the limits of expertise, analysis, validation, and, at times, understanding.

In her 1966 essay "Against Interpretation," the social and cultural critic Susan Sontag made the same point about another realm that mobilizes humanity's capacity for imagination and transformation, namely art. She famously took issue with approaches that subordinate the spiritual power of art to intellectual abstractions, or, as she put it, "the intellect's revenge upon art." Certainly, dying is similar insofar as no observer can adequately do the experience justice. Representing its processes is the prerogative of those who experience it. End-of-life dreams and experiences can therefore not be understood through critical insight and judgment alone, and, in the absence of a subjective perspective of dying, may best be recognized for their effects rather than their workings. Like works of art.

Whereas dreams generally imply that we are lost in sleep, end-of-life experiences pull us into a new, often wakeful, reality. The thirteenth-century Persian mystic poet Rūmī put it best when he stated, in a poem ironically titled "The Dream That Must Be Interpreted," that "Though we seem to be sleeping, there is an inner wakefulness that directs the dream, and will eventually startle us back to the truth of who we are." Although I will continue to maintain, contra Rūmī, that pre-death dreams need not be interpreted to matter, his poetry beautifully represents the moment of recognition when dying and living merge into one. This is when our dreams become reality and end-of-life experiences seem more authentic than the material world that surrounds us.

Some patients withdraw into themselves and are minimally verbal. Others retain an intellectual vitality and a desire to engage with others and express themselves right up to the very end, even when their disease has progressed to the point where they long to die. But most clearly benefit from the therapeutic significance of their pre-death dreams and visions. What should matter, then, is legitimizing dreams rather than exploring their ontological origin (e.g., Freudian or Jungian subconscious, manifestation of a divine world, etc.). For patients, families, and health-care professionals, the therapeutic, existential, and experiential value of these phenomena always comes first.

This value is steeped in transcendence insofar as it points to an existence or experience beyond the physical. It is therefore a state that is often associated with the afterlife. For me, end-of-life experiences represent what happens before, not after, death. I will leave to others the task of debating their repercussions postmortem. Instead, I want to acknowledge the power of this spiritual transformation and transcendence in my patients' lives before they pass on, and show the tremendous difference it makes in caring for them. I want to show the important clinical implications and why we need to take them into account in order to become more literate on the subject of dying.

This being said, it is important to acknowledge that the dying process does bring about a form of spiritual and emotional solace, one that may be rooted in concrete and lived experiences but entails a form of transcendence all the same. Near death, the boundaries between the experiential and the spiritual, the body and the mind, present and past, conscious and unconscious impulses, seem to dissolve to provide a sense of transcendence to a place of blissful comfort and serenity.

All of us get injured or injure for having lived. Yet end-of-life experiences appear to make us whole again, through forgiveness, love, and the return of those we've lost. Old wounds heal as time and distance fade and the span of one's life narrows to what matters. There seems to be a kind of final justice as the end of life excludes those who have caused us harm and embraces those who have nurtured and loved us best. It's fitting perhaps that the circle that gets completed is one of restoration and return to the best parts of having lived.

I used to strive to be the best doctor I could be, while at the same time honoring the spiritual quality of my patients' end-of-life experiences. Now I know that being the best doctor I can be is precisely about recognizing, facilitating, and validating the deeply spiritual nature of such experiences at life's end. Dying is so much more than a physical event. And dying with dignity, just as living with dignity, is so much more of a spiritual than a biomedical process. There is nothing new in this observation. The German poet Rainer Maria Rilke best captured the importance of each individual's expression of meaning in life's final moments when he stated, "I don't want the doctor's death. I want my own freedom." A "good" death has always been about dying on one's own terms and not about the prowess of medical intervention.

It is at the hour of death that people are able to free themselves from old fears and find their way back to a renewed sense of self. This is the whole self with which we lose touch over years of accumulated stressors, expectations, mishaps, and negative emotions, but it is also the self that resurfaces in full force at end of life. During the profound resolution that is enabled by the dying process, patients reconnect with those they have loved and lost, mourned but not forgotten. They relive the unconditional nature of family and familiar connections. They find an alternative to an outside world whose arbitrary demands they once vainly tried to meet.

Western culture's obsession with the dying's final utterances may be born out of these demands, but it is not true to the reality of dying. Famous last words, literary last words, fictional last words . . . popular representations display an intuitive awareness that important things are said and maybe even experienced at life's end, but they seem unable to represent it without hyperbole. They lead us to expect that people's last words matter only if they are poignant and memorable, the capstone of a life's meanings or of a person's insight into them.

But there is no sensationalizing the last stages of life's journey. End-of-life experiences are rarely of a deep philosophical or even religious nature. They don't involve existential questions, exuberant pronouncements, faith-based epiphanies, reckonings, or punch lines. They often simply consist of dreams or visions about everyday events, family, love, even pets.

It is through these reconstituted relationships that the dying often put themselves back together and recover a sense of wholeness. It is precisely a renewed sense of self that our last journey on earth makes possible. In dreams, patients often see themselves as a younger, healthy, and rejuvenated, while paradoxically feeling more like their true self than they ever had. Theologian and psychotherapist Monika Renz refers to this spiritual experience of connectivity as a "loose electrical connection" between self and other. It is a phenomenon that occurs, she explains, in the border region or "liminal space" that opens up between body and mind, consciousness and unconsciousness, at the time of death. Whether it is with one's suppressed self or others, it is exactly this act of connecting, or reconnecting, that patient after patient testifies to experiencing when they describe the effects of their dreams and visions at life's end.

The feeling of a restored bond, between and across lives, is what defined Mary holding and rocking her long-deceased infant on her deathbed or Sierra's mother crawling into her daughter's bed to hold her one last time. It is what helped Sandra, the sixteen-year-old whose grieving parents wanted to spare her the knowledge of her impending death. For her, religion became the lens through which she dreamed of arduously climbing a mountain to reach the angels whose embrace finally provided the relief from suffering she needed. While the journey clearly symbolized death, its outcome evoked togetherness, light, and life.

These examples show the importance of reframing religion at end of life to signify not a rejection but a more expansive understanding of its tenets. At Hospice Buffalo, the medical team knows that working closely with our chaplains and religious representatives is critical to our patients' well-being and happiness. It is now universally understood that the body and the mind impact each other in ways that medicine's exclusive focus on patients' physical symptoms unnecessarily obscures. At end of life, such a compartmentalized view of health is simply not tenable, whether doctors try to maintain it or not. The spiritual and the physical go hand in hand, especially when we seek to ease our patients' transition to their final home.

Despite the inseparable nature of the spiritual and physical aspects of dying, patients paradoxically seldom report religious content in their end-of-life experiences. This book contains several accounts of patients dreaming of religious themes, but the trend is disproportionate when compared to the totality of our data. Other investigators have similarly shown a near absence of religious references in the dreams and visions of the dying. Still, while the paradox is remarkable, it is also hardly the point. After all, family is our first church, and the tenets of faith are love and forgiveness, the very themes of pre-death dreams and visions.

This is an insight that is exemplified in the writings of Kerry Egan, a hospice chaplain in Massachusetts. In her short but powerful piece "My Faith: What People Talk About Before They Die," Ms. Egan explains that she is routinely called to the bedside of dying patients who want to talk, not about God or any big spiritual questions, but about their families and "the love they felt, and the love they gave [or] did not receive, or the love they did not know how to offer, the love they withheld, or maybe never felt for the ones they should have loved unconditionally . . . people talk to the chaplain about their families because that is how we talk about God. That is how we talk about the meaning of our lives. . . . We live our lives in our families: the families we are born into, the families we create, the families we make through the people we choose as friends." In a world where people's success is often measured by the number of relationships they sacrifice along the way, the dreams of the dying help us visualize a world where human relationships define our purpose and our true accomplishment.

For Ms. Egan, not mentioning God directly does not create any conflict between her role as a hospice chaplain and her religious faith because she recognizes God and the teachings of her religion in the love exchanged by family members at the time of death: "If God is love, and we believe that to be true, then we learn about God when we learn about love. The first, and usually the last, classroom of love is the family."

It is true that even patients like Patricia, who worked hard to deny religion, find peace nonetheless. Although she did not "believe in a hereafter [or] believe there's anything over the hill," her pre-death dreams occasioned the same profound transformation of perception as that of people of faith. "So the dreams haven't changed my belief," she stated, "but they've given me comfort." On one of my last visits with her, she even quoted me back to myself. "You mentioned one word," she told me, "and it suits me now. It's *peace*. I really feel peaceful." Is peace not grace by another name?

The writings of Monika Renz similarly testify to the deep spiritual nature of pre-death dreams, regardless of her patients' religious affiliation or lack thereof. Muslim, Jewish, Hindu, Christian, or Buddhist, atheist or agnostic, people are defined by the same human capacity for wholeness at end of life, which Renz describes as a lived experience that "transcends the ego." By that, she means that it moves to a higher context of self that is not limited to the world's conventions and ready-made identities.

At the bedside, I have witnessed again and again the quiet process of peaceful surrender and well-being, the version of grace and spirituality that takes my patients over the threshold of pain and suffering. But if end-of-life dreams are spiritual, they are not so in content so much as in experience. They are spiritual in the manner in which they alter perception and in the sense of well-being they provide. They are spiritual because of the deeply personal process of renewal they trigger in the most secret corners of the self. They are spiritual insofar as they free us from fear and pain and connect us to each other.

There is no detaching human beings from the biological realities of dying. It takes vast courage and resilience to face one's death or the gaze of others on one's disease. My patients' pre-death dreams and visions are a visible manifestation of this inner strength. They help the dying reunite with a more authentic sense of self, with the people they have loved and lost, those who secured them, and those who brought them comfort and peace. Their needs are addressed, whether it is to be guided, reassured, forgiven, or simply loved. Many go to church to get in touch with this kind of reconciliation and inner awareness. Others don't need to.

At the hour of our death, spiritual transformation is no longer external to the self. It happens in the innermost recesses of our being. As we progress toward acceptance, illness and death place us on a spiritual path that ultimately affirms who we are. In chaplain Egan's words, "We don't have to use words of theology to talk about God; people who are close to death almost never do. We should learn from those who are dying that the best way to teach our children about God is by loving each other wholly and forgiving each other fully—just as each of us longs to be loved and forgiven by our mothers and fathers, sons and daughters."

# epilogue

Wherever the art of medicine is loved,
There is also a love of humanity.

—HIPPOCRATES

One of the proudest moments of my life was the day I finally got to put on a white coat and walk into a patient's room as a newly minted physician. In anticipation of this momentous event, I had spent what little money I had on a new suit, tie, and shiny shoes. I was now educated, trained, legitimized, and ready. With all the pride and professionalism I could summon, I entered my first patient's room, introduced myself, and declared in four powerful words, "I am your doctor." The patient looked up and said, "Really? You look like my damn bookie!"

What I learned then and there, and many times since, is that the only point of view that matters is that of the patient. This is what writing this book has been about, the notion that patients who are thought to be silent may in fact be the only people worth listening to.

The assumption that nothing valuable can come from patients in the final weeks and days of life reflects a limited insight into the totality of the dying experience. In many ways, the end-of-life journey is a culmination of an integrative process that distills life into its finest moments. It is about revisiting and re-writing the life scripts we have been handed, whether by chance or by design. Near death is when this process of revision acceler-ates through a distinct vantage point that was not previously available. We all inherit scripts through birth, family, culture, and history that send us down paths not necessarily of our own choosing. Some of them we follow. Others we need to rewrite, sometimes as late as days before death.

My story, like that of many of my patients, is an attempt to rewrite a script in which I had no say. At twelve years old, I nei-ther expected nor accepted the event of my father's death. I met it with pure rage. I had lost a part of me, the sense of purpose and direction he provided, and the image of the man I wanted to become. I did not grieve. I got mad.

Today, my angry and youthful reaction would no doubt be diagnosed as oppositional defiant disorder, but in the 1970s, I was simply labeled "seriously troubled." I went on to get kicked out of one school in seventh grade, and failed eighth grade at another. I became so unmanageable that my mother had no choice but to send me to military-style boarding school. That was in many ways the ideal place for young misfits: picture *Lord of the Flies* with uniforms. But it was no substitute for family and home. I was enrolled for five years, and summers were spent liv-ing and working on a farm. Still, after losing my dad, all punish-ment was relative. Life lessons were lost on me.

My unlikely journey to medical school took an even stranger turn after I started working at Hospice Buffalo. Here, I was confronted by what I had tried to forget ever since childhood: the sight of dying patients with outstretched arms, reaching and calling out to their mothers, fathers, and children, many of whom had not been seen, touched, or heard for decades. I had gone full circle, but this time I could not turn away, because it wasn't about me.

Over time it would be these same patients who helped me rewrite the ending to my dad's story. Where I had once seen only sadness and loss, they helped me recognize something more powerful and life-affirming.

Still, when I lecture on the topic today, there is a point at which I always stumble and go quiet. An audience member will inevitably ask me, "So what do you think this all means?" The question stops me every time. I can go on for days about the perspective of the patient but not about my own. I can testify to how end-of-life experiences affect the dying process, how they work, and how they impact my approach as a doctor, but I grow uncomfortable, even evasive, when asked about what they mean in the grand scheme of things. I sometimes try to get away from the podium with a cursory "Thank you and good-bye" before the inevitable question stumps me.

I remember one day in particular when an older, gruff gentleman at the front of the room intercepted my escape with a more dramatic version of the dreaded question: "So why this entire ruckus about dying?" I paused, and finally came clean about my inability to answer.

The truth is that it was not—and is not—for me to say. I can't begin to speculate on an afterlife or on God's larger plan, which is what many people really want me to talk about. An understanding of what patients experience before death far from qualifies me to comment on what happens after. In fact, I wrote this book precisely because there is something to be said about the dying process outside of its relation to these existential questions. Dying is a mystery in and of itself and not just a harbinger of things to come. Let's not relegate its value to that of a mere prelude to the afterlife. Let's not have it pale by comparison.

The voices and experiences of dying patients matter. My voice and interpretation were never meant to dilute theirs. If anything, it is their experiences that have colored and inspired mine.

So, to the gruff gentleman in the front row, here is a partial answer to the "why the ruckus" question. Dying is more than the suffering we either observe or experience. Within the obvious tragedy of dying are unseen processes that hold meaning. Dying is a time of transition that triggers a transformation of perspective and perception. If those who are dying struggle to find words to capture their inner experiences, it is not because language fails them but because it falls short of the sense of awe and wonder that overcomes them. They experience a growing sense of connectedness and belonging. They begin to see not with their eyes but with their unlocked souls.

For me, what it all means is that the best parts of living are never truly lost. I am reminded of this when elderly patients experience the return of the mother or father they lost in childhood; when soldiers speak of haunting battles; when children talk of dead animals returning to comfort them; and when women cradle babies long lost to their touch. This is when caution vanishes and courage prevails.

I realize then that what matters is not so much what is seen but what is felt.

As poets and writers have reminded us throughout history, love endures. When the end draws near, time, age, and debility vanish to give way to an incredible affirmation of life. Dying is an experience that pulls us together by binding us to those who loved us from the start, those we lost along the way, and those who are returned to us in the end. In the words of Thomas Jefferson, "I find that as I grow older, I love those most, whom I loved first." The dying most often embark on a hopeful journey in which they are embraced one more time by those who once gave their lives meaning, while those who hurt them drift away. Death is also a form of final justice, one in which the scales are balanced by love and forgiveness.

Having witnessed so much death, I can't say that I fully embrace the notion of a "good" death. There is no such thing as a good death, only good people. Death and dying are merely extensions of what came before; we die as we lived. This cannot always be reconciled with happiness or goodness, particularly if the balance of one's life had little to do with either. Although I am often saddened by the tragedy and trauma that so many have endured, I remain amazed by the strength of the human spirit in its endless quest to heal what's harmed or broken. For those denied fulfillment and happiness in life, it may be in that struggle that hope and grace reside.

Before this book ends, I need to go back to how it began. It is simple. When approached, not a single patient or family declined to participate. It is difficult to express the depth of my gratitude, but while it's customary to do so, my thankfulness would actually miss the point. These patients and families did not participate because I asked them; they participated because they wanted to contribute. No matter how ill a person may be, this need to give back is inherent in the struggle to remain connected and human. Even those left behind, the bereaved, fought through tears to give back, in hopes of bringing comfort and understanding to others.

Dying may be isolating and even lonely, but patients often find comfort in spaces where they can continue to express themselves, connect with others, and still matter. Long after the battle to overcome illness is lost, the dying continue to fight, but they are not fighting against, only for and toward. They fight to have relevance, to find meaning—right up until their very last breath. Why else would people, bedridden and fading, find it in themselves to share their stories? Not the embellished versions we typically tell, but the real stuff that comes from having lived and mattered—from hard-felt pains, deep secrets, and distant losses to enduring love and wisdom regained. These moments, measured in days and hours, are not motivated by the possibility of future gain. They constitute a wished-for and self-generated ending.

Illness and tragedy naturally demand that we look inward, an artifact of our fight for survival and our innate resistance against mortality. As sickness begins to overtake the drive to live, there is a shift. The dying continue to cherish life, but not for themselves—for others. They express concern for loved ones, in gestures of kindness and hope, even as they say goodbye. Buried within their stories is the same awe-inspiring message, repeated again and again.

This book evolved from these final good-byes while relaying

stories of hope and grace. So it is with reverence, not just gratitude, that I acknowledge the patients and families who contributed to the writing of these, *their* stories. These are people who had faith that their voices, softened or at times silent, mattered. And that they would still be heard.

# ACKNOWLEDGMENTS

This book arose from the bedsides of patients whose words awed, inspired, and enlightened me.

The experiences of dying patients deserved to be more than a clinical curiosity or described anecdotally. They needed to be told by patients themselves and validated using an evidence-based approach. This book is rooted in studies that were conducted by a talented group of researchers from Hospice Buffalo. This team includes a biochemist, clinicians, and social scientists. My deepest gratitude to Rachel Depner, Kate Levy, Dave Byrwa, and Drs. Scott Wright, Debra Luczkiewicz, James Donnelly, and Sarah Kuszczak. This effort has been led by Dr. Pei Grant, my friend and the wizard behind the curtain.

Thank you also to my friend Jon Hand, who filmed so many of our patients and families. Jon felt more than he could ever capture on film and would often look up from the camera to wipe away his tears. He passed during the writing of this book. Rest in peace, my friend.

My journey from bedside to research to book required a village, a really big village.

With me every step of the way were my hospice colleagues, whose efforts have been tireless, dedication admirable, and compassion unyielding. Our care is at its finest when it is most inclusive of a variety of disciplines, from spiritual care counselors to music therapists. We depend on everyone to provide care in the quiet places where lives, not just disease, need tending.

My gratitude also begins with my friend, medical partner, and mentor, Dr. Robert Milch, a rare and dignified combination of surgeon and social justice warrior. I should probably ask for his forgiveness for going off the rails time and again, but instead I applaud his wisdom in knowing when it was best to simply move the tracks. Thanks to Abby Unger, whose love and support convinced me that there was a story to share in which I had a part to play. This work needed her touch. Special thanks also to Drs. Megan Farrell and John Tangeman for their friendship and for sharing their infinite clinical wisdom.

In 2010, I told a young palliative care fellow, Dr. Anne Banas, that we shouldn't do the original study on the experiences of the dying because "no one would be interested." She replied, "You're nuts." Saying I was wrong doesn't quite cover it, so I can only thank her for her foresight and the passion she has always brought to this work.

I didn't wake up one day and decide to write this book—thankfully my dear friend and agent, Bonnie Solow, did. Having spent my career on the "fringes" of medicine, I never assumed that the words of our patients would reach a receptive audience. Bonnie, however, sought out this project and artfully guided it onto these pages. The patients and families whose words comprise this book deserved a worthy advocate, and she more than answered the call.

It was the fellowship of the horse that brought me together

with my coauthor, Carine Mardorossian, an English professor at the University of Buffalo who boards her horse at my barn. While cleaning stalls, we would often discuss the research and the book's topic, and over several years that conversation led to our partnership in writing this book, a journey of learning, connection, humility, and infinite gratitude. The result is also a powerful testimony to the centrality of the humanities to other fields of knowledge, in this case medicine. I am grateful to Carine for her friendship and her gift for finding the art within the science of medicine.

This book was shaped and guided by early readers—a number of friends from a range of backgrounds and voices, from horse trainers to abstract painters and medical ethicists: Barbara Groh-Wahlstrom, Lynne Kerr, Lonny Morse, Dr. Paul and Noreen Johnson, Tracey Rees, Christy Feightner, Patrick Flynn, Kelley Clem, Sally Green, Shirley Kerr, Jeanne Marohn, and Jane Karol. Thank you for all that you shared and contributed. One of the joys of writing this book has been coming home to my mother rushing to navigate her walker across the room while clutching pages of edits. Your passion has been uplifting.

Thankfully, this book found its rightful home at Penguin Random House. I wish to thank and acknowledge Caroline Sutton, Hannah Steigmeyer, Marie Finamore, Farin Schlussel, Anne Kosmoski, Sara Johnson, and Emily Fisher.

Finally, to my friends and family, particularly my daughters Madison and Bobbie, whose support, understanding, and even forgiveness have been the reassuring constants in a career that often left them shortchanged for time and presence, though never for love.

# NOTES

5. **"It's more than the negative"**: Mitch Albom, *Tuesdays with Morrie* (New York: Doubleday, 2000).

8. **A fear of ridicule:** M. Barbato, C. Blunden, K. Reid, H. Irwin, and P. Rodriguez, "Parapsychological Phenomena Near the Time of Death," *Journal of Palliative Care* 15, no. 2 (1999): 30–7; S. Brayne, C. Farnham, and P. Fenwick, "Deathbed Phenomena and Their Effect on a Palliative Care Team: A Pilot Study," *American Journal of Hospice and Palliative Care* 23, no. 1 (2006): 17–24; Peter Fenwick and Sue Brayne, "End-of-Life Experiences: Reaching Out for Compassion, Communication, and Connection-Meaning of Deathbed Visions and Coincidences," *American Journal of Hospice and Palliative Care* 28, no. 1 (2011): 7–15; S. Brayne, H. Lovelace, and P. Fenwick, "End-of-Life Experiences and the Dying Process in a Gloucestershire Nursing Home as Reported by Nurses and Care Assistants," *American Journal of Hospice and Palliative Care* 25, no. 3 (2008): 195–206.

8. **This widespread inattention further isolates the dying:** Clara Granda-Cameron and Arlene Houldin, "Concept Analysis of Good Death in Terminally Ill Patients," *American Journal of Hospice and Palliative Care* 29, no. 8 (2012): 632–9; L. C. Kaldjian, A. E. Curtis, L. A. Shinkunas, and K. T. Cannon, "Goals of Care Toward the End of Life: A Structured Literature Review," *American Journal of Hospice and Palliative Care* 25, no. 6 (2008): 501–11; William Barrett, *Deathbed Visions* (Guildford, UK: White Crow Books, 2011).

10. **Woman who died in childbirth:** Barrett, *Deathbed Visions*.

11. ***Being Mortal* begins:** Atul Gawande, *Being Mortal: Medicine and What Matters in the End* (New York: Macmillan, 2014).

11. ***When Breath Becomes Air:*** Paul Kalanithi, *When Breath Becomes Air* (New York: Random House, 2016).

12. **"To get the 'I' out of the experience":** Alan Watts, *The Wisdom of Insecurity: A Message for an Age of Anxiety* (New York: Vintage Books, 1951).

13. **"I will not say that one should *love* death":** Rainer Maria Rilke, "Letter to Countess Margot Sizzo, January 6, 1923," in *Letters of Rainer Maria Rilke, vol. 2, 1910–1926*, trans. Jane Bannard Greene and M. D. Herter Norton (New York: W. W. Norton, 1947), 316.

21. **Half of all dying patients visit:** A. Smith, E. McCarthy, E. Weber, I. S. Cenzer, J. Boscardin, J. Fisher, and K. Covinsky, "Half of Older Americans Seen in Emergency Department in Last Month of Life; Most Admitted to Hospital, and Many Die There," *Health Affairs* 31, no. 6 (2012): 1277–85.

22. **"Today, healing is replaced with treating":** Bernard Lown, *The Lost Art of Healing: Practicing Compassion in Medicine* (New York: Ballantine, 1999).

28. **"The secret for caring for the patient":** Francis Peabody, "The Care of the Patient," *Journal of the American Medical Association* 88, no. 12 (1927): 877–82.

32. **Clinically based papers on the subject:** Karlis Osis, *Deathbed Observations by Physicians and Nurses* (New York: Parapsychology Foundations, 1961); Karlis Osis and Erlendur Haraldsson, *At the Hour of Death* (Norwalk, CT: Hastings House, 1997); P. Fenwick, H. Lovelace, and S. Brayne, "Comfort for the Dying: Five Year Retrospective and One Year Prospective Studies of End of Life

Experiences," *Archives of Gerontology and Geriatrics* 51, no. 2 (2010): 173–9; A. Kellehear, V. Pogonet, R. Mindruta-Stratan, and V. Gorelco, "Deathbed Visions from the Republic of Moldova: A Content Analysis of Family Observations," *Omega* 64, no. 4 (2011–2012): 303–17; Brayne, Lovelace, and Fenwick, "End-of-Life Experiences and the Dying Process"; M. Lawrence and E. Repede, "The Incidence of Deathbed Communications and Their Impact on the Dying Process," *American Journal of Hospice and Palliative Care* 30, no. 7 (2012): 632–9; Brayne, Farnham, and Fenwick, "Deathbed Phenomena and Their Effect on a Palliative Care Team."

35. **Patients with delirium:** American Psychiatric Association, *Diagnostic and Statistical Manual of Mental Disorders*, fifth edition (Washington, DC: American Psychiatric Association, 2013).

35. **These experiences differ most from hallucinations or delirium:** Brayne, Lovelace, and Fenwick, "End-of-Life Experiences and the Dying Process"; James Houran and Rense Lange, "Hallucinations That Comfort: Contextual Mediation of Deathbed Visions," *Perceptual and Motor Skills* 84, no. 3, pt. 2 (1997): 1491–504; April Mazzarino-Willett, "Deathbed Phenomena: Its Role in Peaceful Death and Terminal Restlessness," *American Journal of Hospice and Palliative Care* 27, no. 2 (2010): 127–33; Fenwick and Brayne, "End-of-Life Experiences."

42. **Large-scale examination of the experiences of dying patients:** Osis and Haraldsson, *At the Hour of Death*.

43. **They too used surveys and case analyses:** Peter Fenwick and Elizabeth Fenwick, *The Art of Dying: A Journey to Elsewhere* (London: Bloomsbury, 2008).

43. **To document end-of-life experiences as told by patients:** C. Kerr, J. P. Donnelly, S. T. Wright, S. M. Kuszczak, A. Banas, P. C. Grant,

and D. L. Luczkiewicz, "End-of-Life Dreams and Visions: A Longitudinal Study of Hospice Patients' Experiences," *Journal of Palliative Medicine* 17, no. 3 (2014): 296–303.

49. **In another study, we identified distinct thematic categories:** C. Nosek, C. W. Kerr, J. Woodworth, S. T. Wright, P. C. Grant, S. M. Kuszczak, A. Banas, D. L. Luczkiewicz, and R. M. Depner, "End-of-Life Dreams and Visions: A Qualitative Perspective from Hospice Patients," *American Journal of Hospice and Palliative Care* 32, no. 3 (2015): 269–74.

69. **Confirmed the role that pre-death dreams and visions play in post-traumatic growth:** K. Levy, P. C. Grant, R. M. Depner, D. J. Byrwa, D. L. Luczkiewicz, and C. W. Kerr, "End-of-Life Dreams and Visions and Posttraumatic Growth: A Comparison Study," *Journal of Palliative Medicine* (forthcoming).

71. **18 percent of end-of-life dreams among our study patients were distressing in nature:** Levy et al., "End-of-Life Dreams and Visions and Posttraumatic Growth."

76. **With a description of both comforting and upsetting dreams:** Jan Hoffman, "A New Vision for Dreams of the Dying," *New York Times*, February 2, 2016.

98. **Shocking adoption of the tenets of American eugenics by state schools:** Michael D'Antonio, *The State Boys Rebellion* (New York: Simon & Schuster, 2005).

154. **"Medical science has rendered obsolete centuries of experience":** Gawande, *Being Mortal*.

185. **"This is the essence of magic":** Franz Kafka, *The Diaries of Franz Kafka, 1910–1923* (New York: Knopf Doubleday, 1988).

187. **The moving tribute his wife wrote:** Kalanithi, *When Breath Becomes Air*, epilogue.

194. **Effect of end-of-life dreams on the grieving family:** T. Morita, A. S. Naito, M. Aoyama, A. Ogawa, I. Aizawa, R. Morooka, M. Kawahara, et al., "Nationwide Japanese Survey About Deathbed Visions: 'My Deceased Mother Took Me to Heaven,'" *Journal of Pain and Symptom Management* 52, no. 5 (2016): 646–54.

194. **Influenced their overall grief journey:** P. C. Grant, R. M. Depner, K. Levy, S. M. LaFever, K. Tenzek, S. T. Wright, and C. W. Kerr, "The Family Caregiver Perspective on End-of-Life Dreams and Visions During Bereavement: A Mixed Methods Approach," *Journal of Palliative Medicine* (forthcoming).

208. **Suggest that it is not always imperative for patients to interpret their pre-death dreams:** Kelly Bulkeley and Patricia Bulkley, *Dreaming Beyond Death: A Guide to Pre-Death Dreams and Visions* (Boston: Beacon Press, 2005).

213. **Mobilizes humanity's capacity for imagination and transformation:** Susan Sontag, *Against Interpretation* (New York: Farrar, Straus and Giroux, 1966).

214. **"Though we seem to be sleeping":** Jalāl al-Dīn Rūmī, *The Essential Rumi*, trans. Coleman Barks (San Francisco: Harper, 1995).

217. **spiritual experience of connectivity as a "loose electrical connection":** Monika Renz, *Hope and Grace* (London: Jessica Kingsley, 2016).

219. **"We live our lives in our families":** Kerry Egan, "My Faith: What People Talk About Before They Die," *Belief* (blog), CNN.com, January 28, 2012, http://religion.blogs.cnn.com/2012/01/28/my-faith-what-people-talk-about-before-they-die.

# INDEX

sleep, and dying process, 35, 40, 48, 51, 61, 66, 146, 178, 214

Sonny and Joan, story of, 127, 132–36, 139, 140, 142, 200–201

Sontag, Susan, 213–14

spiritual transformation in dying, 4, 5, 9, 13, 18, 28, 59, 69, 120, 167, 168, 200, 213, 215, 216, 217, 218, 220, 221

*See also specific stories*

SS *James L. Ackerson*, 58

*State Boys Rebellion, The* (D'Antonio), 98, 100

Stinson, John's story, 189, 210

"Stitches" (Mendes), 157–58

stress-induced cardiomyopathy (broken-heart syndrome), 129

subjective experience of dying, 2, 3, 4, 9, 10, 11, 12, 28, 31, 32, 35, 194, 214

suicide, 64, 74

supernatural, 202

Susan (Beverly and Bill's daughter), story of, 134, 135, 136, 137–38

symptom demands of illness, 25–26

takotsubo cardiomyopathy (broken-heart syndrome), 129

Tammy and Sierra, story of, 6, 189–93, 195, 218

Tangeman, John, 175, 176–77

Tedx Buffalo talk, Christopher Kerr, 11, 19

"terminal business," 64

themes, end-of-life experiences, 49–51, 183

therapeutic opportunity from end-of-life experiences, 69, 106

Thomas, Dylan, 173

Thomas (Doris's father), 99

Tim, story of, 53–55

"tiny little thing" called love, 128, 142

Tom, story of, 1–2, 8, 13–14, 17, 48

Tony (Sandra's friend), 161, 162, 163

total pain (Saunders), 87

transcendence in dying, 120, 215

transcendental realm, 209–10

transcending the ego (Renz), 220

transformative power of end-of-life experiences, 46, 72, 82, 111, 168, 213, 215, 221, 226

*See also specific stories*

travel theme, 47, 50, 183

*Tuesdays with Morrie* (Albom), 5

uniqueness of end-of-life experiences, 3, 44, 59–60, 111, 134, 181, 185, 210

*See also specific stories*

University of Buffalo, 32, 37, 42

USS *Texas*, 58

Vaagen, Gerd, story of, 175–77

Valentine's Day, 130, 131

waiting for particular date or visitor before dying, 60–61

"waiting for them" theme, 6, 41, 49–50, 60, 74, 81

wakefulness and end-of-life experiences, 40, 43, 51, 178, 214

Walter E. Fernald State School ("Fernald"), 100–102, 103

war experiences, 33, 57–59, 65, 123, 124, 138, 175, 176, 189, 210

war metaphor of terminal illness, 145, 152

Watts, Alan, 12

*When Breath Becomes Air* (Kalanithi), 11, 187–88